STROKE

Advances in
Prevention & Treatment of

CEREBROVASCULAR
DISEASE

2017 Report

A Special Report published
by the editors of *Heart Advisor*
in conjunction with
Cleveland Clinic

Stroke: Advances in the Prevention & Treatment of Cerebrovascular Disease

Consulting Editor: Efrain D. Salgado, MD, Director, Stroke Center, Cleveland Clinic Florida—Weston

Contributing Editor: Holly Strawbridge
Group Directors, Belvoir Media Group: Diane Muhlfeld, Jay Roland
Creative Director, Belvoir Media Group: Judi Crouse

Publisher, Belvoir Media Group: Timothy H. Cole

ISBN: 978-1-879620-84-1

To order additional copies of this report, or copies of *Coronary Artery Disease* or *Heart Failure*, or for customer service questions, please call 877-300-0253; write Health Special Reports, 535 Connecticut Avenue, Norwalk, CT 06854-1713; or go to www.Heart-Advisor.com/HealthSpecialReports.

This publication is intended to provide readers with accurate and timely medical news and information. It is not intended to give personal medical advice, which should be obtained directly from a physician. We regret that we cannot respond to individual inquiries about personal health matters.

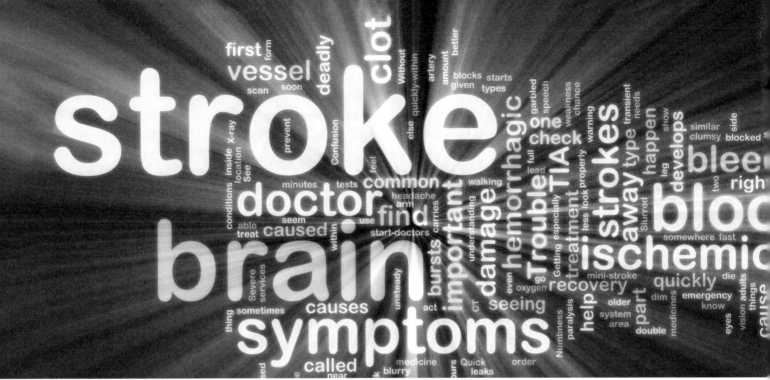

NEW FINDINGS

TABLE OF CONTENTS

TABLE OF CONTENTS

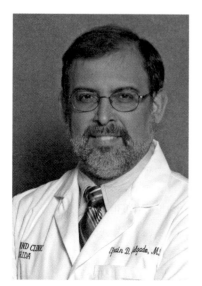

Efrain D. Salgado, MD
Director, Stroke Center
Cleveland Clinic Florida Weston

Every year, approximately 795,000 people in this country suffer a stroke, and about 129,000 of them die. This makes "brain attack" the fifth most common cause of death in the United States.

The encouraging news is that stroke deaths have declined 19 percent since 2003, largely because people have taken steps to control risk factors such as hypertension, diabetes, smoking, and high cholesterol. Today, an estimated 6.6 million stroke survivors age 20 and older are living in the United States. Many, unfortunately, are disabled: 10 percent of stroke survivors require care in a nursing home or long-term care facility, 40 percent experience moderate-to-severe impairments that require special care, and 25 percent recover with minor impairments. Only 10 percent recover almost completely.

That's why it is so important to know how to lower your risk for stroke. It's equally important to know what happens if you have a stroke, and what treatment and rehabilitation options are available to you.

About 14 percent of stroke survivors have a second stroke within a year. If you have survived a stroke, it is in your best interest to do everything you can to prevent another. Once you are out of the hospital, it will be up to you to reduce your risk factors. You need to understand why you are taking any medications you have been prescribed and know how to recognize symptoms that may indicate an evolving stroke, so you know when to call 911.

If you have not had a stroke, but your doctor has told you that you are at high risk of having one, you are still fortunate. Use the information in this book to lower your risk, and follow your doctor's advice and recommendations.

Efrain D. Salgado, MD
Director, Stroke Center
Cleveland Clinic Florida Weston

Advances in the Prevention and Treatment of Cerebrovascular Disease

A stroke comes "out of the blue." It happens when you least expect it. And when you have a stroke, it can change your life in ways you never imagined.

In this report, you'll learn what actually happens when a stroke occurs. You'll also learn what causes strokes. Although a stroke is sudden and severe, it may be the result of an ongoing medical condition that could be treated to reduce the risk by as much as 50 to 80 percent. This report will explain how. You'll also learn about medications your doctor may prescribe, and about advanced interventions that can help people at high risk for stroke lower their risk. You'll learn how strokes are treated—including exciting new advances in emergency care— and how advances in rehabilitation programs after a stroke are improving recovery.

About Cleveland Clinic

Cleveland Clinic in Cleveland, Ohio, is a not-for-profit, multispecialty academic medical center that integrates clinical and hospital care with research and education. Cleveland Clinic was founded in 1921 by four physicians who had a vision of providing outstanding patient care based on the principles of interdisciplinary cooperation, compassion, and innovation.

Cleveland Clinic has been consistently recognized as one of the best hospitals in America by *U.S. News & World Report* since the magazine began rating hospitals in 1990. Every year since 1994, Cleveland Clinic has been ranked the top hospital in the United States for heart care. The Sydell and Arnold Miller Family Heart & Vascular Institute's more than 130 physicians, practicing in the Robert and Suzanne Tomsich Department of Cardiovascular Medicine and departments of Cardiothoracic Surgery and Vascular Surgery, provide patients with access to state-of-the-art cardiovascular care.

For more than five decades, Cleveland Clinic physicians and scientists have earned worldwide recognition for major contributions to the understanding of hypertension, atherosclerosis, diabetes, hypercholesterolemia, blood-clotting mechanisms, and other factors that influence cerebrovascular disease.

The Cerebrovascular Center, including the Joint Commission-certified Comprehensive Stroke Center at Cleveland Clinic's main campus and a network of eight Primary Stroke Centers throughout Northeast Ohio, manages one of North America's highest stroke-related patient volumes, with more than 3,200 stroke discharges and 1,100 surgical/ interventional procedures annually.

Cleveland Clinic's multidisciplinary Neurological Institute includes more than 300 medical, surgical, and research specialists dedicated to the diagnosis and treatment of adult and pediatric patients with neurological and psychiatric disorders. *U.S. News & World Report's* "America's Best Hospitals" survey has consistently ranked Cleveland Clinic's neurology/

Pioneering Cleveland Clinic Neurological Contributions

- Digital subtraction angiography, developed in conjunction with two other centers
- Non-surgical photon therapy for the treatment of arteriovenous malformations
- Brain stress test to identify patients at risk for stroke
- Skull-base and circulatory arrest technique for aneurysm treatment
- Familial incidence of cerebral aneurysms in polycystic kidney disease confirmed
- New concepts for treating life-threatening, stroke-related brain swelling
- First national trial of surgical decompression for stroke-related brain swelling
- American College of Radiology guidelines for diagnosis and treatment of cerebrovascular disease
- Extracranial/intracranial bypass surgery
- Organization of hypothermia trials for stroke
- Trial of mechanical revascularization following embolic stroke (lead clinical site)
- First clinical trial of hypothermia for acute ischemic stroke (COOL AID)
- First randomized trial of carotid stenting with emboli prevention (SAPPHIRE, lead clinical site)
- One of a handful of organizations in the country using the Pipeline Embolization Device, allowing for the endovascular treatment of large or giant wide-necked intracranial aneurysms
- One of two institutions pioneering Mobile Stroke Treatment Units in the U.S.
- Only Mobile Stroke Treatment Unit to use telemedicine services to manage patients before they arrive in the hospital

neurosurgery programs among the top 10 in the nation, and its pediatric neurology/neurosurgery program among the top in the nation.

Cleveland Clinic led the first trial comparing carotid stenting with carotid endarterectomy in the treatment of stroke, and the first randomized, multicenter trial demonstrating the clinical efficacy of intra-arterial thrombolysis in patients with acute stroke of less than six hours' duration caused by middle cerebral artery occlusion. These are only two of many innovations that have earned Cleveland Clinic an international reputation as the leader in cerebrovascular, as well as cardiovascular, care.

Cleveland Clinic neurological specialists provide comprehensive care for more stroke patients than almost any other physicians in North America. This high volume of patients, along with the physicians' skills and their use of evidence-based medicine, have produced a team capable of managing the most seriously ill, complex patients.

ABOUT THE BRAIN ATTACK

When blood flow is interrupted for more than a few seconds, the neurons (brain cells) begin to malfunction. If blood flow is not restored quickly, the neurons begin to die. This is why immediate medical evaluation and treatment is absolutely essential for people who are experiencing symptoms of a stroke.

A stroke is what happens when blood flow to part of the brain is interrupted in a way that injures or kills brain cells. There are three ways this can happen:

1. A blood vessel can become blocked, preventing blood from flowing through it.
2. Blood pressure can suddenly drop, preventing blood from reaching the brain.
3. A blood vessel can burst, spilling blood into surrounding brain tissue.

The way blood flow to the brain is interrupted defines the two major types of stroke: ischemic and hemorrhagic (see Box 1-1, "Ischemic vs. Hemorrhagic strokes").

BOX 1-1

Ischemic vs. Hemorrhagic Strokes

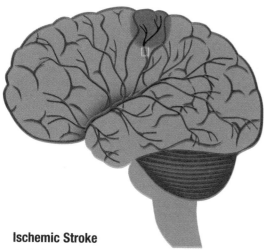

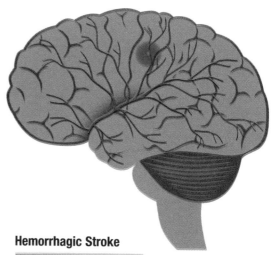

Ischemic Stroke

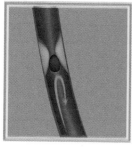

An ischemic stroke is caused by a blockage of blood vessels, which leads to a lack of blood flow to the affected area.

Hemorrhagic Stroke

A hemorrhagic stroke is caused by a rupture of blood vessels and leakage of blood into the brain.

BOX 1-2

Ischemic Stroke

About 87 percent of all strokes are ischemic. These strokes most often occur when an artery bringing blood to the brain becomes blocked, and blood flow stops. Less frequently, a sudden, severe drop in blood pressure causes an ischemic stroke.

Brain cells (neurons) rely on a constant stream of blood supplying oxygen and nutrients to operate normally. When blood flow is interrupted for more than a few seconds, the neurons begin to malfunction. If blood flow is not restored quickly, the neurons begin to die. This is why immediate medical evaluation and treatment is absolutely essential for people who are experiencing symptoms of a stroke.

There are two types of ischemic strokes:

Embolic Stroke

Sometimes a clot that develops elsewhere in the body—typically the heart, aorta, or carotid arteries in the neck—breaks off and travels in the bloodstream to the brain. This type of clot is called an embolus. When an embolus lodges in a brain artery, stopping blood flow, it causes an embolic stroke.

Thrombotic Stroke

When a clot (thrombus) develops in a narrowed part of an artery—typically from fatty buildup in the arteries (atherosclerosis) of the brain or neck—the result is a thrombotic stroke. This type of stroke comprises about 50 percent of all strokes. A thrombotic stroke is further differentiated as a large-vessel or small-vessel thrombosis, depending on the size of the artery in which the thrombus occurs. A small-vessel thrombotic stroke deep within the brain is also called a lacunar stroke. These strokes can cause unique symptoms (see Box 1-2, "About Lacunar Strokes").

How Ischemic Strokes Are Categorized

Ischemic strokes are categorized according to the severity and duration of symptoms:

▶ Transient ischemic attack (TIA). A TIA is a sudden, transient episode of neurological dysfunction caused by a lack of blood flow to part of the brain. It passes without causing permanent

About Lacunar Strokes

The symptoms of a lacunar stroke depend on which part of the brain is affected. The most common symptom is weakness or paralysis on one side of the body.

Some lacunar strokes cause sensory symptoms, such as numbness, burning, tingling, freezing, pain, or any number of odd sensations that occur only on one side of the body. Motor defects and sensory symptoms may occur together.

Lacunar strokes are more common in men than women, and are often associated with hypertension, older age, smoking, or diabetes.

Lacunar strokes that damage the thalamus deep in the brain can result in chronic pain that patients describe as a burning or aching sensation. If medication fails to relieve this pain, a treatment called deep brain stimulation (DBS) may help.

damage to the brain. TIAs typically last no more than 20 minutes or so. They are sometimes called mini-strokes, but they are actually "transient strokes." If you have a TIA, you are at higher risk for having stroke in the next two to 90 days. It's urgent that you be evaluated immediately to determine the cause of the TIA, so steps can be taken to prevent a full-blown stroke. Because it's very hard to tell the difference between a stroke and a TIA until the TIA resolves, it's wisest to treat a TIA as a medical emergency by calling 911.

▶ Progressing or evolving stroke. This is a stroke in the process of occurring. The sooner you get to an emergency department for stabilization and treatment, the better your outcome will be. If the stroke is treated quickly, you may have no lasting deficit or disability. However, some treatments are only effective if they are administered within the first few hours of symptom onset.

▶ Completed stroke. This is a cerebral infarction, and it means the stroke was severe enough and lasted long enough to kill a portion of brain tissue. Irreversible deficit, disability or death is likely. Doctors consider a stroke to be completed when the elapsed time from the start of symptoms is too long to permit any effective intervention.

Hemorrhagic Stroke

When a weakened artery in the brain ruptures, the result is a hemorrhagic stroke. Blood flowing into the brain compresses the tissue and kills brain cells.

The two types of hemorrhagic strokes are defined by their location within the skull. About 75 percent of hemorrhagic strokes (13 percent of all strokes) occur within the brain itself. These are called intracerebral hemorrhages. In the other 25 percent the bleeding occurs in the space between the brain and the skull. These are known as subarachnoid hemorrhages (see Box 1-3, "Intracerebral and Subarachnoid Hemorrhagic Strokes," on page 13).

Hemorrhagic strokes can be devastating: About 40 percent of hemorrhagic strokes that occur within the brain itself (intracerebral hemorrhages) cause death.

About 10 to 15 percent of people who suffer a subarachnoid

BOX 1-3

Intracerebral and Subarachnoid Hemorrhagic Strokes

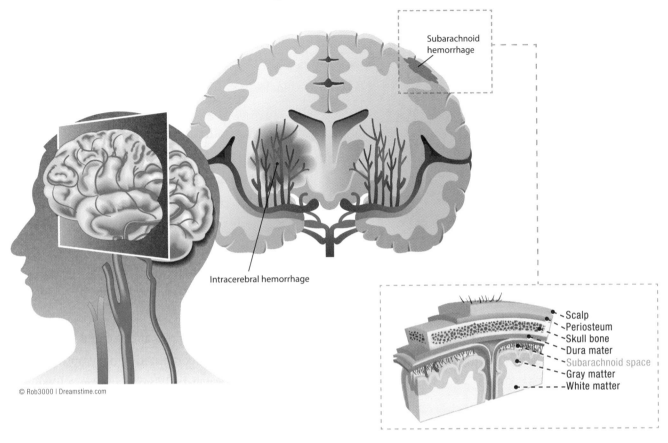

Subarachnoid hemorrhage

Intracerebral hemorrhage

© Rob3000 | Dreamstime.com

Scalp
Periosteum
Skull bone
Dura mater
Subarachnoid space
Gray matter
White matter

hemorrhage from a ruptured aneurysm die before reaching the hospital; 40 percent die within the first week; and 50 percent die within the first six months.

The most common cause of a spontaneous subarachnoid hemorrhage is a ruptured aneurysm. An aneurysm is a balloon-like outpouching from a weakened area of the wall of an artery, typically at the base of the brain. Aneurysms are present at birth. Cerebral aneurysms carry a higher risk of rupture in patients with a family history of ruptured aneurysms, and in those who currently smoke, have a large aneurysm, or suffer from high blood pressure.

Stroke Is an Emergency!

When a stroke occurs, some brain function is usually lost. Just how much is lost depends on the type of stroke, its location, and how quickly the stroke is treated (see Box 1-4, "Good Evidence That Faster Treatment Improves Outcomes").

NEW FINDING BOX 1-4

Good Evidence That Faster Treatment Improves Outcomes

Neurologists use the saying, "Time is brain," to underscore the importance of rapid treatment for ischemic stroke. Now researchers in the MR CLEAN trial, conducted in the Netherlands, have confirmed that the faster a blockage is opened and blood flow is restored, the better the chance of a favorable outcome with little or no disability. In fact, the researchers found that the risk of a bad outcome increased six percent for every hour treatment was delayed.

JAMA Neurology, December 21, 2015

BOX 1-5

Know the Symptoms of Stroke

If you experience a stroke, call 911 immediately, then call your doctor. Calling your doctor first may delay lifesaving treatment. The quicker you receive treatment, the better the chance your brain function can be preserved. It's better to err on the safe side by requesting emergency care immediately if you suspect you might be having a stroke. Don't delay, even if the symptoms disappear.

Common Symptoms of Stroke:

- Sudden numbness, weakness, or paralysis, typically affecting only one side of the body, including or excluding the face
- Sudden difficulty swallowing, chewing, or moving the tongue
- Sudden trouble seeing in one eye or both eyes
- Sudden confusion
- Sudden difficulty speaking or understanding
- Sudden trouble walking or loss of coordination

Symptoms Can Also Include Sudden:

- Sensation of spinning (vertigo)
- Double vision: seeing two objects when there is only one
- Tendency to look toward or away from the side of the body affected by weakness or partial or total paralysis
- Inability to assemble, construct, or draw objects
- Unawareness or neglect of the neurological deficit or the inability to recognize body parts
- Inability to make decisions or lack of willpower
- Urinary incontinence
- Excruciating headache that may be accompanied by vomiting and a stiff neck
- Seizures
- Aggressive behavior: shouting obscenities, hitting, biting and becoming agitated
- Loss of consciousness
- Death

Stroke symptoms often affect only one side of the body. Because each side of the brain controls the movement of the opposite side of the body, a stroke that occurs in the right side of the brain may cause weakness and/or numbness on the left side of the body, and vice versa.

- When a clot blocks the right middle cerebral artery, which feeds the area of the brain controlling voluntary movement and receiving sensory input for touch, pain, and heat and cold, symptoms may include paralysis, weakness, numbness, or loss of vision on the left side of the body.
- If the stroke affects the right side of the brain, symptoms may include the inability to recognize the left side of the body.
- When a clot blocks the left middle cerebral artery, symptoms will affect the right side of the body and the ability to speak and understand language.

Depending on what part of the brain is affected and how severe the stroke is, a single symptom or combination of symptoms may occur with varying degrees of severity. Women are more likely than men to experience non-traditional symptoms that may not be understood as a stroke, such as confusion, disorientation, or loss of consciousness. Because these symptoms are easily misunderstood, they are less likely to trigger a 911 call than traditional symptoms.

Although most strokes occur with little or no warning, immediate medical attention is crucial to increasing the chance of recovery without any neurological or functional deficit. Knowing the symptoms of stroke could save your life (see Box 1-5, "Know the Symptoms of Stroke"). Make sure your family and companions know the signs and symptoms as well. If you experience a stroke, call 911 immediately, then call your doctor. Calling your doctor first may delay lifesaving treatment. The quicker you receive treatment, the better the chance your brain function can be preserved. It's better to err on the safe side by requesting emergency care immediately if you suspect you might be having a stroke. Don't delay, even if the symptoms disappear.

The emergency treatment for ischemic stroke is administration of a powerful clot-busting medication called intravenous tPA. It must be given within 4½ hours after symptoms begin, keeping in mind that the earlier it is administered within that time period, the better the chances of a favorable outcome. There may be some exceptions; researchers are still trying to find the best way to identify these individuals. Until this is known, it's important to try to note the time symptoms begin, or make sure someone else can tell emergency personnel when the stroke likely occurred.

Some people awaken in the morning to find they suffered a stroke overnight, and the time it occurred cannot be determined. Because the time of stroke onset is unknown, these patients are generally not candidates for tPA. However, some data suggests it may be relatively safe and effective, if patients meet certain criteria (see Box 1-6, "Treating Wake-Up Stroke May Be Feasible After All"). Research is underway to determine whether imaging might better be able to determine which patients with "wake-up strokes" are most likely to benefit from clot-busting therapy.

If you suffer a stroke, your chances for a good outcome are best if you travel to the hospital by ambulance. An ambulance is the fastest way to get to the hospital, and emergency medical services (EMS) personnel can begin initial assessment and management on the way to the hospital, saving valuable time. This increases your chance of getting the treatment you need within the window of opportunity. Ambulance personnel know which hospitals are designated stroke centers, and they will notify hospital staff, who will be ready to act as soon as you arrive.

Driving while you are experiencing a stroke puts you and other motorists at risk, especially if your symptoms worsen. Strokes are unpredictable, so there is no way to know the severity or duration of your symptoms.

When you arrive at the Emergency Department of your local hospital, the doctors will work fast to confirm you are having a stroke, and if so, whether your stroke is ischemic or hemorrhagic. This information is essential, because the treatments for these strokes are very different.

Prognosis

The extent of your disability (if any) will be determined after the stroke has ended and your condition has been stabilized. The

Treating Wake-Up Stroke May Be Feasible After All

About 30 percent of stroke victims arrive at the hospital without anyone knowing what time the stroke occurred. In many cases, these patients simply awakened with symptoms. Physicians hesitate to give these patients tPA, for fear it may cause more harm than good. The results of a 2016 study called MR WITNESS may put these fears to rest. The researchers found a variety of MRI imaging modalities could be used to obtain a score that allowed the patients to safely receive tPA, so long as they had been seen without symptoms and apparently healthy 4.5 to 24 hours earlier.

International Stroke Conference, February 2016

length of time you will need to recover from a stroke will depend on its severity. Fortunately, about 50 to 70 percent of stroke survivors are able to regain functional independence. Others are permanently disabled to various degrees.

Although a stroke can occur at any age, about two thirds of people hospitalized for stroke are age 65 and older. Unfortunately, up to 50 percent of older adults who develop one or more symptoms of stroke do not seek emergency medical care. Older patients tend to have additional medical problems that affect their ability to recover from a stroke, so recognizing the warning signs and taking quick action increase the chances of preventing or at least surviving a stroke.

The risk of dying from stroke varies with the type of stroke and increases with age. The prognosis after hemorrhagic stroke is grim. With ischemic stroke, about nine percent of patients aged 65 to 74, 13 percent of patients aged 74 to 84, and 23 percent of those age 84 and older die within 30 days.

Sometimes, dramatic measures are taken to decrease the risk of death—for example, temporarily removing part of the skull to allow for brain swelling. Although this procedure can halve the risk of death, a hefty percentage of patients survive only to experience severe disabilities.

HOW STROKES HAPPEN

In this chapter, we will discuss your brain's "plumbing," and show you what ischemic and hemorrhagic strokes look like.

Cerebrovascular disease is the term used for any disease affecting the blood vessels of the brain: "Cerebro" refers to the brain and "vascular" pertains to blood vessels (see Box 2-1, "Views of the Brain"). Cerebrovascular diseases include those caused by arteries blocked by a blood clot, bleeding in or around the brain caused by a ruptured blood vessel, and any change in the brain's blood vessels that alters the normal flow of blood. Loss of blood flow to the brain for even a short time can damage or kill brain cells. The more brain cells that are affected, the greater the likelihood the stroke will cause permanent disability or death.

BOX 2-1

Views of the Brain

Cerebrum and cerebellum: The **cerebrum** is the largest part of the brain. It contains your memory, and it is responsible for your sensory perception (vision, smell, touch, hearing, and taste), voluntary movements, higher thought functions (thinking, planning, organizing, and problem solving), and the emotions and behavior that shape your personality. The **cerebellum** controls voluntary and involuntary movement, including balance.

Involuntary body function: Most involuntary bodily functions, such as breathing, heart rate, blood pressure, body temperature, and sleeping, are controlled by smaller regions of the brain located at the top of the spinal cord. These include the medulla oblongata, pons, thalamus, hypothalamus, amygdala, and pituitary gland.

Right and left hemispheres: The brain is divided into the left and right hemispheres, which have the same structures. Although similar in appearance and anatomy, the two hemispheres process information in different ways, and one side is dominant. In general, the left side is the logical side, while the right side is the creative, artistic side.

Body signals: The brain receives and sends information to the body through nerves, most of which enter the brain through the spinal cord at the bottom of the brain. Several so-called "facial nerves" relay signals back and forth directly to the brain, not through the spinal cord. The optic nerve from your eyes, for example, does not enter the brain through the spinal cord, but through the optic chiasm.

Major Lobes
- Frontal lobe
- Parietal lobe
- Occipital lobe
- Temporal lobe
- Cerebellum
- Brain stem

Smaller Regions of the Brain

Located at the top of the spinal cord: Amygdala, hypothalamus, medulla oblongata, pituitary gland, pons, and thalamus.

Brain Functions
- Association
- Coordination
- Emotion
- Eye movement
- Higher mental functions
- Hearing
- Language comprehension
- Sensory
- Smell
- Somatosensory association
- Speech
- Vision
- Voluntary motor function

Lateral View

Sagittal View

Inferior View

Superior View

LEFT

RIGHT

Hemispheres

BOX 2-2

Circulatory System

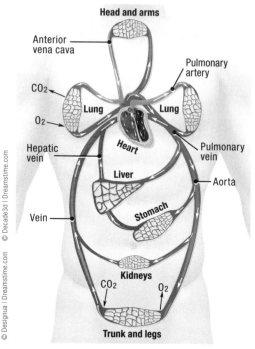

To make a complete circuit, blood enters and leaves the heart twice.

First, the right side of the heart pumps blood carrying carbon dioxide, a waste product of cell metabolism, through the pulmonary arteries to the capillaries of the lungs, where carbon dioxide is exchanged for oxygen.

The freshly oxygenated blood returns to the left side of the heart via the pulmonary veins.

The left side of the heart pumps the oxygenated blood throughout the body, distributing other nutrients and transporting other metabolic waste products to the kidneys in the process. In the capillaries, the blood releases oxygen to the tissues and organs and absorbs carbon dioxide.

Two major veins return the deoxygenated blood to your heart: the superior vena cava, which drains the head and arms, and the inferior vena cava, which drains the torso and legs.

The arteries have thicker walls and are more elastic than veins, because they must stretch to accommodate the full force of the blood pumped out of the heart. Veins have thinner walls, because they don't carry blood under the same pressure.

Your Circulatory System

Your circulatory system delivers blood to all organs and tissues of your body. Your heart is the pump, and your blood vessels are the plumbing. It's a closed system: Blood pumped from the heart eventually returns to the heart, where it is sent to the lungs for oxygen and back to the heart to be pumped through the system again (see Box 2-2, "Circulatory System"). The blood vessels that deliver oxygenated blood from the heart to your tissues and organs are called arteries; those that return oxygen-depleted blood to your heart are called veins. (Because veins are not usually involved in common cerebrovascular diseases, they will not be discussed here).

Arteries are largest in diameter where they leave the heart and become smaller and smaller until they turn into capillaries. Capillaries are only large enough for red blood cells to flow through in single file. They deliver oxygen to the body's tissue in exchange for carbon dioxide. After blood passes through the capillaries, it enters the veins, which return it to the heart.

Your Brain's Plumbing

You have large arteries that lead from the heart to the brain, as well as a network of arteries inside the brain. The artery affected by a stroke is critical to diagnosis and treatment and may influence your prognosis, particularly if you have suffered a hemorrhagic stroke.

Blood flow to the brain begins when oxygenated blood leaves the left side of the heart and enters the aorta, the biggest artery in the body. Just after the aorta leaves the heart, it branches into three arteries that supply blood to the upper part of the body, including your brain (see Box 2-3, "Arteries of the Head and Neck," on page 19). The first branch is called the brachiocephalic trunk, which divides into the right common carotid artery and right subclavian artery. The right vertebral artery branches from the right subclavian artery. The second branch from the aorta is the left common carotid artery. The third branch is the left subclavian artery, from which the left vertebral artery originates. The common carotid and vertebral arteries send blood to the head and brain, while the right and left subclavian arteries supply blood to the arms.

The Carotid Arteries

Just below the level of the jaw, the common carotid arteries branch into the internal and external carotid arteries. The internal carotid artery goes to the brain, and the external carotid artery goes to the skin and muscles of the head and neck. The internal carotid arteries are responsible for about 80 percent of the blood flow to the brain: The remainder is delivered by the two vertebral arteries. After branching off the subclavian arteries, the vertebral arteries turn toward the spine and follow to the back of the brain, where they enter through holes in the vertebrae. Thus, the brain receives blood from four arteries: the left and right internal carotid arteries, and the left and right vertebral arteries.

Arteries of the Brain

In every individual, the paths of the smaller arteries and veins differ, but the basic patterns of blood flow through the brain are usually similar.

The internal carotid arteries and vertebral arteries enter the skull and run through the subarachnoid space between the brain and the skull. The vertebral arteries join together near the pons (part of the brainstem) to form a single artery called the basilar artery (see Box 2-4, "Arteries of the Brain," on page 20). The basilar artery runs the length of the pons and has several tiny branches that nourish the brainstem. The anterior inferior cerebellar arteries and superior cerebellar arteries are larger branches that supply the cerebellum. The basilar artery terminates in cerebral arteries that supply the visual cortex (sight center).

Within the Internal Carotid Arteries

Meanwhile, after entering the skull, both internal carotid arteries divide into three arteries known as the anterior cerebral, middle cerebral, and posterior communicating arteries. The anterior cerebral arteries send blood to the front of the cerebrum. Before they do, however, they join together to connect the left and right sides of the brain's circulation via an anterior communicating artery. The two posterior communicating arteries run toward the back of the brain and connect with the posterior cerebral arteries

BOX 2-3

Arteries of the Head and Neck

External carotid artery

Internal carotid artery

Vertebral artery

Common carotid artery

Brachio-cephalic trunk

Sub-clavian artery

Aorta

© Sebastian Kaulitzki | Dreamstime.com

branching off the basilar artery. These connections create a continuous loop known as the circle of Willis.

The circle of Willis is important because it provides collateral circulation. When you turn your head from side-to-side or up and down, the arteries in your neck stretch and flex. In the process, they may become compressed, which restricts blood flow. You don't faint when this happens, because the circle of Willis provides collateral blood flow. Likewise, when you turn your head as far as possible to one side, one of your internal carotid arteries is compressed. Without the circle of Willis, this would stop blood flow to one side of your brain. However, the circle of Willis ensures that blood from the other internal carotid artery is distributed throughout the brain.

Collateral circulation also provides an alternate path for blood to reach any part of the brain, should one of the major arteries become obstructed. If an internal carotid artery is blocked, for example, the other major arteries partly compensate for the loss of blood flow. Other cerebral arteries may also connect, providing collateral circulation to other parts of the brain. This varies among individuals, however. In fact, a complete circle of Willis may occur in only 40 percent of people. The more collateral

BOX 2-4

Arteries of the Brain

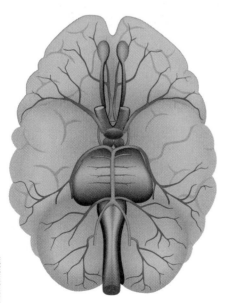

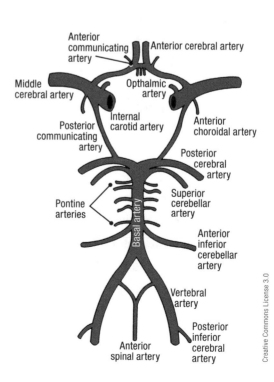

Blood flowing to the brain enters the skull through the two internal carotid arteries and the two vertebral arteries.

These four arteries are connected by way of the basilar artery, formed by the fusion of the two vertebral arteries and the circle of Willis.

The circle of Willis is made up of the anterior and posterior communicating arteries, portions of the anterior and posterior cerebral arteries, and the end of the basilar artery, where it divides into the two posterior cerebral arteries.

circulation you have, the better your chance of surviving a stroke without severe deficits.

Causes of Strokes

Ischemic strokes are generally the result of a blockage caused by cardiovascular disease (atherosclerosis), but they can also be caused by a clot (embolism) that forms in the heart or aorta, breaks away, and becomes lodged in a brain artery. People with atrial fibrillation, valve disease, and artificial heart valves are at risk for these so-called emboli. Other rare conditions can also cause an ischemic stroke (see Box 2-5, "Rare Causes of Ischemic Strokes").

Certain medications, including ranibizumab (Lucentis)

BOX 2-5

Rare Causes of Ischemic Strokes

Less than five percent of ischemic strokes are caused by unusual or rare conditions or diseases. These include dissections, hypercoagulable states, vasculitis, and systemic hypotension.

Dissections

Arteries are comprised of several different types of cells that allow them to stretch, contract, and relax. These include layers of muscle cells and elastic tissues. An arterial dissection occurs when a tear in the innermost layer allows blood to flow between these layers, separating them. A dissection is usually confined to a small area of an artery, but since the blood has no place to go and comes in contact with surfaces that stimulate blood clotting, it clots. When a dissection occurs in an artery leading to the brain, a stroke may happen. Dissections are most often caused by blunt trauma to the head and neck or chiropractic manipulations of the neck. Because younger people are more active in sports, about five to 20 percent of ischemic strokes in patients under 45 years of age are caused by dissections, compared to about one to 2.5 percent of all ischemic strokes in the general population.

Hypercoagulable States

Under normal conditions, blood is fluid and unlikely to clot. Certain diseases however, cause blood to clot when ordinarily it would not. When this happens, the blood is said to be hypercoagulable. Inherited deficiencies in certain blood proteins involved in blood clotting can be responsible, as can pregnancy; oral contraceptive use in women who have high blood pressure, smoke, or have migraines; obesity; cancer; chemotherapy; lupus erythematosus; and certain kidney diseases. In a hypercoagulable state, blood clots may form spontaneously, and if they flow into an artery of the brain, cause a stroke.

Vasculitis

This condition is characterized by inflammation of the blood vessels. Many forms of vasculitis are treatable. A common feature, however, is the tendency for blood to clot as it flows through an affected artery. When vasculitis affects arteries in the brain or arteries leading to the brain, a stroke may occur.

Systemic Hypotension

This sudden, significant drop in blood pressure can be caused by life-threatening heart rhythm disturbances that cause blood flow to stop.

BOX 2-6

Plaque Formation in the Arteries

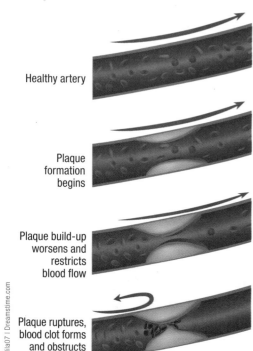

Healthy artery

Plaque formation begins

Plaque build-up worsens and restricts blood flow

Plaque ruptures, blood clot forms and obstructs blood flow

© Alila07 | Dreamstime.com

for macular degeneration and COX-2 inhibitors for arthritis pain, may raise the risk of stroke. Your physician will weigh the benefits of these drugs against the possible risk before prescribing them.

Causes of hemorrhagic stroke include high blood pressure, cerebral amyloid angiopathy, ruptured aneurysms, vascular malformations, head trauma, brain tumors, blood thinning medications, and other medical and neurological conditions that either weaken cerebral blood vessels or thin the blood.

Atherosclerosis

Atherosclerosis is a progressive disease that damages the arteries and affects how well they function. Unfortunately, it may not cause symptoms until a stroke occurs. The good news is that many risk factors for atherosclerosis have been identified, and there's a lot you can do to minimize your risk (see Chapter 3).

In atherosclerosis, cholesterol and other substances are deposited within the arterial wall, and certain types of cells begin to grow and divide, forming plaques. In some cases, these plaques become so large they may restrict or block the flow of blood. They can also erupt or break apart. Plaque promotes local clot formation, and if the clot grows so large that it halts blood flow, the result is a thrombotic stroke. If it breaks apart, pieces of plaque and blood clot may flow into the bloodstream as emboli. When emboli lodge in a smaller artery and obstruct blood flow, an embolic stroke occurs.

Plaque Formation

Plaques likely start at a young age and may take years—even decades—to grow. Most people are unaware they have growing plaques, because symptoms do not appear until 70 percent or more of the artery's interior channel (lumen) is blocked (see Box 2-6, "Plaque Formation in the Arteries").

Plaques develop in three phases. The first is called "initiation." The lining of arteries (endothelium) is a smooth, inert surface that blood flows across. High cholesterol levels, high blood pressure, toxins in cigarette smoke, and other factors can damage the endothelium and stimulate the development of atherosclerosis.

Injured endothelial cells interact with white blood cells, which are part of the body's defense against infectious organisms such as bacteria. White blood cells attack the invaders, help heal the injuries, and rid the body of cells that may have been irreparably injured or killed. This process, called inflammation, is a natural response to injury. It paves the way for the growth of new cells and tissues to replace those that were killed or damaged. Certain white blood cells help ensure that this process occurs in an orderly manner. But to get to the injury they must leave the blood and enter the tissues, which requires crossing the endothelium. Injured endothelium responds by becoming sticky to attract white blood cells.

If the risk factor that caused the injury is removed, the endothelial cells will heal and return to their normal behavior. But if the injury keeps occurring—if you continue smoking or allow your blood pressure or cholesterol to remain high, for example—white blood cells continue to be recruited and stick to the artery wall at the site of injury.

Plaque Growth

Cholesterol impacts plaque development. Cholesterol is a type of fat made by your liver and absorbed from digested food. Your body needs only a tiny amount of cholesterol to make hormones, bile, and vitamin D. If unused cholesterol is not excreted, the body deposits it on artery walls.

Cholesterol molecules are wrapped in protein-covered particles that move easily through the bloodstream. These are called lipoproteins. There are four main types of lipoproteins:
- Low-density lipoproteins (LDL)
- High-density lipoproteins (HDL)
- Very-low-density lipoproteins (VLDL)
- Chylomicrons primarily containing triglycerides

Low-density and high-density lipoproteins contain high concentrations of cholesterol, and chylomicrons are another dangerous fat.

LDL, VLDL, and chylomicrons carry fats from the gut and the liver throughout your body to meet the cells' metabolic needs. HDL carries fats to the liver, which prepares it for removal from the body. That's why HDL-cholesterol is called "good," and

Hard, Asymptomatic Plaques Rarely Cause Stroke

When hard plaques build up in the carotid arteries, it would be reasonable to assume you'll suffer a stroke if the plaque obstructs blood flow. But that may not be the case. Researchers followed more than 3,600 patients with carotid artery disease, but no symptoms of stroke. Over time, only nine percent developed total blockages, and only one patient had a stroke. Three more developed a stroke an average of three years later. Why? The researchers explained that collateral circulation through the circle of Willis (see page 20) helps maintain blood flow through the cerebrum, even when one or both carotid arteries are blocked.

JAMA Neurology, September 21, 2015

LDL-cholesterol is called "bad." LDL plus HDL and 20 percent of your triglycerides equals total cholesterol, which is measured after fasting. (Chylomicrons and VLDL appear only after a meal).

When the different lipoproteins exist in proper proportion, they are not a health risk. However, when total cholesterol or LDL-cholesterol levels rise, or the amount of HDL-cholesterol drops, the body starts depositing cholesterol in the arteries. Although triglycerides do not accumulate in arteries like cholesterol does, abnormally high levels of triglycerides are also associated with an increased risk of stroke or heart attack.

Plaque Maturation

At least four things begin to happen as the plaque enlarges. First, some of the white blood cells inside the fatty streak begin to die, forming what doctors call a "necrotic core." Second, the muscle cells of the artery wall begin to grow over the necrotic core. Third, blood cells called platelets begin to stick to the injured endothelium and facilitate the formation of small blood clots on the surface of the plaque. Platelets are an essential component of blood clotting in arteries. These disc-shaped cells are much smaller and flatter than red blood cells. Normally, they circulate without doing much. But when they sense an injury that causes bleeding, they clump together to stop it by forming a plug. They also present a sticky surface that attracts actual blood clots formed from circulating proteins. As the plaque enlarges, platelets and blood clots get mixed in with the cells covering the necrotic core to form a fibrous cap. The cap is delicate and prone to rupture, releasing its contents into the bloodstream. This is a highly dangerous situation.

Plaque Hardens

In the fourth stage of plaque development, certain cells in the slowly developing plaque deposit calcium inside the plaque—a process called "hardening of the arteries." By the time a plaque develops to this point, it contains many different types of cells, both living and dead, lots of cholesterol and lipoproteins, pieces of old blood clots, and calcium. Thus, it has become a "complex" plaque. These plaques tend to grow slowly and may or may not produce symptoms (see Box 2-7, "Hard, Asymptomatic Plaques Rarely Cause Stroke").

The Heart-Brain Connection

Atherosclerosis can affect almost any artery in the body. Symptoms vary, depending on the organ fed by that artery. When atherosclerosis affects arteries supplying blood to the brain or inside the brain, the result is a stroke. When atherosclerosis affects the arteries supplying blood to the heart muscle (coronary artery disease, or CAD), the result is a heart attack. The same disease process can affect the arms and legs (peripheral arterial disease, or PAD) or the kidneys (renovascular disease).

Patients with atherosclerosis in one site are at increased risk of having atherosclerosis elsewhere. If you have had an ischemic stroke, or have experienced symptoms of a transient ischemic attack (TIA) that indicate increased risk for stroke (see Box 2-8, "Symptoms of a Transient Ischemic Attack"), you have a 20 to 40 percent chance of having CAD. In fact, two to five percent of ischemic stroke survivors have a fatal heart attack less than 90 days after their stroke. If you are under the age of 60 and have a TIA, your risk of having a heart attack is 15 times that of a healthy person your age.

Similarly, CAD is a risk factor for stroke, since patients with CAD may also have cerebrovascular disease. In addition, they are at increased risk for strokes caused by blood clots forming in the heart and traveling to the brain. While about 47 percent of all deaths from cardiovascular disease are due to CAD, about 16 percent are due to stroke.

Aortic Arch Atheroma

In patients with atherosclerosis, the aortic arch can be a source of blood clots. This is known as aortic arch atheroma, and it tends to affect older patients with high blood pressure. Although the arch itself is large and not likely to become blocked with plaque, atherosclerotic plaques that form in this region are prone to breaking off and traveling toward the brain.

It is now clear that plaques in the aortic arch should be treated medically. However, the optimal medical regimen is unclear. Antiplatelet therapy and statin therapy are recommended. Most patients are not candidates for surgical treatment of the aortic arch, due to a greatly increased risk

BOX 2-8

Symptoms of a Transient Ischemic Attack

- About 15 percent of strokes are preceded by a transient ischemic attack (TIA). TIAs are characterized by symptoms of stroke that last a short time, then disappear as quickly as they appeared.

- A TIA is a warning sign that your immediate risk of stroke is high. After a TIA, the risk of stroke within 48 hours is three to 10 percent, and nine to 17 percent within 90 days. About 12 percent of people die from stroke (per diagram below) within one year of experiencing a TIA.

- Those who survive have a 10-year stroke risk of 19 percent, and a combined 10-year risk of stroke, heart attack, or vascular death of 43 percent.

- Because it is often impossible to tell the difference between a TIA and a stroke, the symptoms should be treated as an emergency.

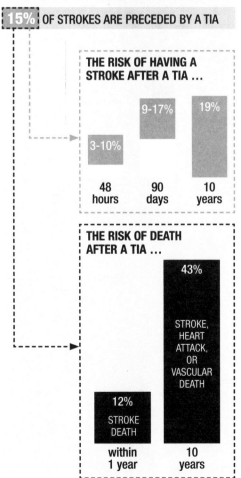

15% OF STROKES ARE PRECEDED BY A TIA

THE RISK OF HAVING A STROKE AFTER A TIA …

48 hours	90 days	10 years
3-10%	9-17%	19%

THE RISK OF DEATH AFTER A TIA …

within 1 year	10 years
12% STROKE DEATH	43% STROKE, HEART ATTACK, OR VASCULAR DEATH

BOX 2-9

Diseases of the Mitral Valve

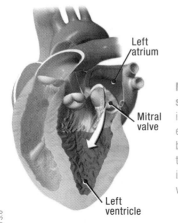

Left atrium

Mitral valve

Left ventricle

Mitral valve stenosis impedes the emptying of blood from the left atrium into the left ventricle.

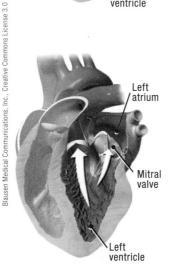

Left atrium

Mitral valve

Left ventricle

Mitral regurgitation allows blood to flow backward into the left atrium.

Blausen Medical Communications, Inc., Creative Commons License 3.0

of a stroke occurring during the operation. Lowering blood pressure, lowering cholesterol, and stopping smoking are most important in preventing these plaques from growing.

Heart Valve Disease

Diseases of the mitral valve, which connects the left atrium and left ventricle, are associated with increased risk of ischemic stroke. Mitral stenosis and mitral regurgitation account for most of these strokes. A bacterial infection known as infective endocarditis can cause plaque and other debris to slough off, resulting in an embolic stroke. Fortunately, treatment with antibiotics can greatly reduce the risk.

The mitral valve has two leaflets (also called cusps or flaps), which open inward when pressure is higher in the left atrium than in the left ventricle (see Box 2-9, "Diseases of the Mitral Valve"). As pressure builds in the contracting ventricle, the leaflets slam shut, preventing blood from being pumped backwards into the atrium. In a condition called mitral stenosis, the calcified leaflets become rigid, preventing them from opening well. The edges of the leaflets can also fuse, reducing the size of the opening through which blood flows.

As stenosis begins to impede the emptying of blood from the left atrium into the left ventricle, blood backs up in the pulmonary circulation. The lungs become fluid-filled and congested, causing shortness of breath. After several years of mitral stenosis, it's also common for atrial fibrillation or other atrial arrhythmia to develop.

In mitral regurgitation, the leaves of the mitral valve fail to form a tight seal when the ventricle contracts, allowing blood to flow backwards into the atrium and backing up in the pulmonary circulation. The symptoms are similar to those of mitral stenosis.

About two-thirds of all cases of mitral stenosis and one-third of all cases of mitral regurgitation are caused by rheumatic heart disease, which is now rare in the U.S. Mitral regurgitation may also occur after a heart attack, particularly if the papillary muscles attached to the mitral and tricuspid valves are affected. Mitral regurgitation may also occur in heart failure, particularly when the left ventricle enlarges from dilated cardiomyopathy.

Atrial Fibrillation

Atrial fibrillation is a heart rhythm disturbance (arrhythmia) originating in the upper chambers of the heart (atria). When atrial fibrillation lasts for more than several days, it is said to be persistent. It may also last for a short time and revert to normal spontaneously, without any treatment. This kind of "paroxysmal" (intermittent) atrial fibrillation is not uncommon, and may occur following surgery or exercise, or in people who are emotionally stressed or inebriated. Regardless of type, atrial fibrillation increases ischemic stroke risk (see Box 2-10, "Atrial Fibrillation and Stroke").

Atrial fibrillation affects four percent of people age 60 and older, and its incidence increases with age. Nine percent of people age 80 and older have atrial fibrillation. One-third of people age 85 and older with atrial fibrillation will have a stroke, compared with only 16.7 percent of people in this age group without the arrhythmia. Atrial fibrillation most often occurs in people with high blood pressure, coronary artery disease, heart valve disease, or cardiomyopathy.

When the cause of stroke is not immediately clear, the doctor may recommend a 30-day heart-rhythm monitor or an insertable cardiac monitor. The latter device is implanted under the chest skin, where it can monitor the heart's electrical signals for as long as necessary. Information downloaded from the device will reveal whether the patient is having intermittent or paroxysmal atrial fibrillation. If so, a blood thinner such as warfarin, factor Xa inhibitor, or direct thrombin inhibitor can be prescribed to prevent another stroke.

Atrial Fibrillation and Stroke Risk

Untreated atrial fibrillation increases the risk for ischemic stroke five-fold. That's because uncoordinated, poor pumping action of the heart may cause blood to pool in some areas of the left atrium and form a clot. Most of these clots form in a sac called the atrial appendage. From there, the clot may become dislodged and flow into the left ventricle, where it is pumped through the aortic valve into the aorta and on through the common carotid or vertebral arteries, internal carotid arteries, and finally into one of the smaller cerebral arteries, where it lodges, causing an ischemic stroke.

BOX 2-10

Atrial Fibrillation and Stroke

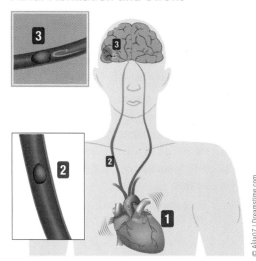

© Ailia07 | Dreamstime.com

A blood clot can form during atrial fibrillation (1). The blood clot travels in the bloodstream (2), and blocks an artery in the brain (3), causing a stroke. This type of stroke is an ischemic embolic stroke.

BOX 2-11

How Blood Pressure is Measured

Blood pressure is reported as two numbers. The top number (systolic) is the pressure when the heart beats. The bottom (diastolic) is the blood pressure between heartbeats.

Blood pressure is measured in millimeters of mercury, abbreviated as mm Hg (Hg is the atomic symbol for mercury), even though most modern blood pressure measuring devices (sphygmomanometers) no longer use mercury-filled tubes.

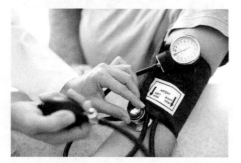

To measure blood pressure, a cuff is placed around the upper arm and inflated. When fully inflated, the cuff compresses the blood vessels in the arm, stopping blood flow. As the technician slowly releases air from the inflated cuff, pressure falls. With the help of a stethoscope on the inside of the elbow, the technician records the systolic blood pressure when it is strong enough to push blood through the constricted artery. Diastolic blood pressure is recorded when the cuff is deflated enough to allow unrestricted blood flow of blood. At this point the artery goes silent, and the technician can no longer hear the blood flowing.

Hypertension

According to the American Heart Association, 80 million U.S. adults have hypertension, meaning their blood pressure is 140/90 mm Hg or higher. Normal or healthy blood pressure is currently defined as less than 120/80 mm Hg (see Box 2-11, "How Blood Pressure is Measured"). Pressures between 120/80 and 140/90 mm Hg are called "pre-hypertension." Hypertension greatly increases the risk of stroke, heart attack, heart failure, and kidney failure. It also increases the risk of second stroke among stroke survivors. Widely fluctuating blood pressure may be an even greater danger.

Most people with hypertension have essential hypertension, also known as primary hypertension—meaning the high blood pressure is a disease in itself, rather than being caused by something else. High blood pressure can progress for years without causing symptoms, yet is easy to identify at a regular checkup.

Hypertension is dangerous because increased pressure and stress on the blood vessels causes arteries to age faster, making them more likely to rupture and cause hemorrhagic stroke or develop fatty plaques, which increases the risk of ischemic stroke. Hypertension appears to increase the risk of "silent strokes" deep in the brain by as much as 60 percent.

Most hypertension-related hemorrhages in the brain are spontaneous and occur most commonly in the small arteries located deep in the brain, in the basal ganglia, cerebellum, and pons. A hemorrhage in another part of the brain is likely due to a different cause, although hypertension may play a role.

Patent Foramen Ovale

A patent foramen ovale (PFO) is a hole between the right and left atria. Before birth, the hole enables blood from the umbilical cord to flow from the right atrium to the left atrium, bypassing the lungs, which have not yet begun to work. At birth, the hole usually closes permanently, but in about 20 to 25 percent of people it remains open or patent (pronounced PAY-tent). PFO is associated with stroke in people younger than age 50, and is found during autopsy in about 40 percent of patients who die from ischemic stroke at a young age.

A PFO is not simply a hole, but a hole with a flap (see Box 2-12, "Patent Foramen Ovale"). After the umbilical cord is cut, the flap normally closes and fuses to the edge of the opening to form a solid wall. When the flap remains open, blood flows from the right atrium into the left atrium when the pressure on the right side is greater than on the left. This can occur when a person coughs, sneezes, or strains on the toilet. The danger is that an embolus on the right side of the heart will pass to the left side, where it is eventually pumped to the brain and causes a stroke. The source of these emboli is thought to be blood clots in leg veins. Older patients with PFO and a condition called deep vein thrombosis (DVT) are at increased risk of stroke.

Most people with a PFO never notice any symptoms or suffer a stroke. Despite the increased risk of stroke conferred by PFO, repairing asymptomatic PFOs discovered accidentally may actually further increase the risk of stroke. Surgeons speculate that the stitches used to secure the flap may attract clots, more than doubling the risk of leaving the flap alone. In patients who have suffered a stroke that may be caused by a PFO, repairing the PFO is no better than medical therapy with blood-thinning drugs at preventing another stroke.

Obstructive Sleep Apnea

When you sleep, the muscles in your neck relax. In some people, this causes their throat to collapse, slowing or temporarily halting their breathing. When this happens repeatedly throughout the night, it is called obstructive sleep apnea (OSA). People with OSA may be unaware they stop breathing, but other people are very aware, because OSA causes heavy snoring interrupted by periods of silence that end with a gasp. Poor quality sleep may cause the person to feel excessively sleepy during the day.

Studies have shown OSA increases the risk of a fatal or nonfatal stroke and heart attack. Some patients with OSA are overweight and have excess fat in the neck. In these people, losing weight may cause OSA and its associated risks to disappear. In other patients, OSA appears to be associated with nasal obstruction and the shape of the tongue, airway, palate, and jaw.

BOX 2-12

Patent Foramen Ovale

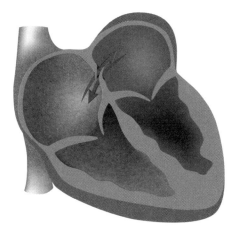

A patent foramen ovale is a hole between the right and left atria that normally closes shortly after birth. When it fails to close, it significantly increases the risk for stroke at a young age.

Aneurysms

Aneurysms form in weakened areas of an artery wall. As the wall weakens, even normal blood pressure can cause it to balloon out (see Box 2-13, "Enlarging Aneurysm").

Aneurysms most often form in arteries located at the base of the brain, particularly where the arteries divide, such as in the circle of Willis. It is believed that many aneurysms begin early in life and enlarge slowly until they suddenly rupture many years later. Smoking and hypertension increase the risk of rupture. About 20 percent of people with one aneurysm have several aneurysms. A person with a parent or sibling who has had an aneurysm is at increased risk.

Aneurysms may also form in smaller arteries that branch off the major arteries in the subarachnoid space. These microaneurysms usually cannot be seen on imaging. Most researchers believe that hypertension and smoking contribute to the development of microaneurysms.

A burst aneurysm is the most common cause of a spontaneous subarachnoid hemorrhagic stroke. When this occurs, the

BOX 2-13

Enlarging Aneurysm

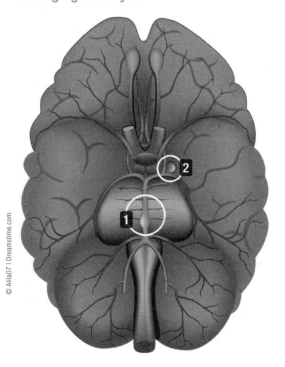

© Alila07 | Dreamstime.com

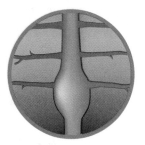

1 Fusiform Aneurysm

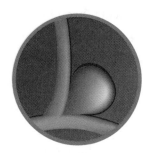

2 Saccular Aneurysm

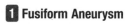

A saccular cerebral aneurysm accounts for the majority of intracranial aneurysms. They're also the most common cause of non-traumatic subarachnoid hemorrhage. It's also called a berry aneurysm because of its shape.

subarachnoid space begins to fill with blood. Symptoms include a sudden, intense headache, neck pain, and nausea or vomiting. If the pressure builds up rapidly and compresses parts of the brain, it may cause loss of consciousness or death. About half of all subarachnoid hemorrhage patients who arrive at the hospital alive die within 30 days. More than half of those who survive suffer major neurologic deficits or other complications.

Non-ruptured aneurysms are typically discovered incidentally on brain imaging performed for another condition. It is difficult to predict which aneurysms are prone to rupture. Physicians consider factors such as the size of the aneurysm, family history, and use of tobacco products in their decision to offer preventive treatment. This is often weighed against the risk of surgical treatment. As aneurysms grow, they may press on certain nerves or areas of the brain, disrupting their normal function. This may result in dilation of a pupil or loss of a light reflex in the eye, other vision defects, or focal pain in the head or neck.

Other Causes

Other causes of hemorrhagic stroke include cerebral amyloid angiopathy, arteriovenous malformations, certain blood-clotting diseases, brain tumors and head trauma, hyperthyroidism, and cocaine abuse. Even something as common as breathing air filled with dust and soot appears to increase stroke risk. The culprit is fine-particle pollution, which comes primarily from motor vehicle exhaust, power plant emissions, and other operations that involve the burning of fossil fuels.

Cerebral Amyloid Angiopathy

In some people, a protein called beta-amyloid accumulates in the small arteries throughout the brain (cerebral amyloid angiopathy). This is the same protein seen in Alzheimer's disease. Affected arteries become weaker and more brittle, making them more likely to rupture. It is not known why beta-amyloid accumulations cause hemorrhage in some individuals and Alzheimer's disease in others.

Some patients may have multiple hemorrhages over a period

of months or years. Some small ones may be asymptomatic ("silent").

Cerebral amyloid angiopathy may occur in more than one-third of people age 60 and older. Unfortunately, there is no treatment for it. The risk of spontaneous hemorrhage can be reduced by managing hypertension and avoiding drugs that prevent blood from clotting.

Arteriovenous Malformations

Arteriovenous malformations (AVM) are congenitally abnormal blood vessels that grow between arteries and veins in the brain. A direct shunt between an external carotid artery branch and a vein is called an intracranial dural arteriovenous fistula (AVF). Both are prone to rupture and spill blood into the brain. AVMs and AVFs can be tiny or large. Some AVMs never cause symptoms, while others may cause headaches, seizures and, if they burst, hemorrhagic stroke. These vascular malformations are rare in the general population and often go undetected unless a patient develops symptoms or undergoes brain imaging for another reason.

Blood Diseases, Blood-Clotting Deficiencies

Blood diseases and blood-clotting deficiencies that increase the risk of a hemorrhagic stroke include leukemia, aplastic anemia, and thrombotic thrombocytopenic purpura (TTP). Certain inherited disorders that cause abnormally long bleeding times, such as hemophilia, are also associated with increased risk of brain hemorrhage. Drugs that inhibit blood clotting may also increase the risk of a cerebral hemorrhage.

Brain Tumors

Brain tumors that originate in the brain or have metastasized from tumors located elsewhere in the body may cause intracerebral hemorrhage. Sometimes a hemorrhage is the first indication a brain tumor is present. As tumors grow, they stimulate the growth of new arteries and veins to reinforce their blood supply. These new arteries may not be fully formed and may be weaker and more prone to rupture from ordinary blood pressure fluctuations or hypertension.

Head Trauma

A serious injury to the head may cause an artery in the brain to rupture. Any time a person exhibits unexplained neurologic deficits following an accident or sports injury, an intracerebral hemorrhage may be responsible.

Hyperthyroidism

An overactive thyroid has been shown to increase the risk of stroke by 44 percent in adults under age 45. Although hyperthyroidism may not be directly responsible, various mechanisms associated with hyperthyroidism—including hypercoagulability, hypofibrinolysis, endothelial dysfunction, and atrial fibrillation—make hyperthyroidism a risk factor.

Factors That Increase Risk

Race

Blacks are at particularly high risk for stroke. According to the American Heart Association's Heart Disease and Stroke Statistics—2016 Update, black men and women have double the risk of a first stroke than whites. The reasons are not clear. Some of the increased incidence may be explained by untreated risk factors, such as high blood pressure or diabetes.

Gender

Women are at greater risk for stroke than men. Each year, about 55,000 more women than men suffer a stroke. Although women share many risk factors with men, much of the increased risk is due to factors unique to women:

- The risk of stroke rises three-fold during pregnancy and remains high for six weeks after giving birth.
- Stroke is more likely to occur in women who experience infections or preeclampsia, or who have other risk factors for stroke, such as hypertension or diabetes.
- Women who naturally enter menopause before age 42 have twice the risk of ischemic stroke.
- After menopause, hormone replacement therapy with estrogen and progestin increases the risk of stroke by 31 percent in women with an intact uterus. After hysterectomy, treatment with estrogen alone increases the risk of stroke

Migraine With Aura Associated With Cardioembolic Stroke

Doctors have known that migraine with aura increases the risk of ischemic stroke. But only recently, the subtype of stroke has been identified. In the 12,844 adults aged 45 to 64 in the Atherosclerosis Risk in Communities (ARIC) study, 817 ischemic strokes occurred between 1987 and 2012. Patients who suffered migraine with aura had more than double the risk of those without this form of migraine. Then, researchers discovered that these adults were more likely to have a cardioembolic stroke—the kind that starts with a clot in the heart—than a thrombotic or lacunar stroke. Further studies are needed to determine whether a treatment as simple as an aspirin a day, or aspirin plus a daily statin, can reduce the risk of stroke in patients with migraine with aura.

International Stroke Conference, February 2016

by 39 percent. The risk with low-dose estrogen patches is lowest.

- Migraine with aura is associated with ischemic stroke in younger women, especially if they smoke or take oral contraceptives (see Box 2-14, "Migraine With Aura Associated With Cardioembolic Stroke").
- Women with atrial fibrillation or high blood pressure have a significantly higher stroke risk than men with these risk factors.

Evidence-based recommendations for what women can do to lower their stroke risk can be found in 2014 guidelines issued by the American Heart Association. To read the full report free of charge, please visit http://bit.ly/1uxdEYV.

Common Infections

Several studies have identified an increased risk of stroke among individuals recently exposed to common viruses and bacteria. It is not yet known whether aggressive treatment to eradicate these pathogens lowers the risk of stroke. How these infections increase the risk or "trigger" strokes is not known, but it is suspected they cause chronic low-level inflammation in the blood vessels.

While we all get sick from viral and bacterial infections from time to time and usually recover in a few days, these pathogens can cause lasting damage. One study found that cumulative exposure to five common pathogens increases the risk of stroke: the viruses herpes simplex 1 and 2 and cytomegalovirus, and the bacteria *Chlamydia pneumoniae* and *Helicobacter pylori*. Another study found that ocular shingles caused by the herpes zoster virus, the same virus that causes chickenpox, more than quadrupled the risk of stroke.

Although the risk of stroke in children is low—about five in 100,000—research has shown that a significant percentage of children who have a stroke had an infection in the days leading up to the event. The risk was highest within a few days of developing an infection and essentially disappeared a month after the infection. Researchers said their findings shouldn't raise alarms, as childhood infections are common. However, they suspect a genetic component common to the young stroke patients. Further study is needed to reach a more definitive conclusion.

Geographic Location

The risk for stroke varies by geographic region, with the highest rates of stroke in the southeastern United States, an area known as the "stroke belt." It includes North Carolina, South Carolina, Georgia, Tennessee, Mississippi, Alabama, Louisiana, and Arkansas (see Box 2-15, "Stroke Belt"). The risk of dying from stroke in the stroke belt is about 20 percent higher than in the rest of the United States.

At least part of the difference is explained by the fact that people living in the Southeast have higher rates of high blood pressure and diabetes. The Southern-style diet of foods rich in grease (think fried chicken, fish and potatoes), salt (bacon, ham), and sugar (sweet tea) may also increase the risk of stroke. Studies have shown people who eat a Southern-style diet six times a week have a 41 percent greater chance of having a stroke than someone who indulges once a month.

BOX 2-15

Stroke Belt

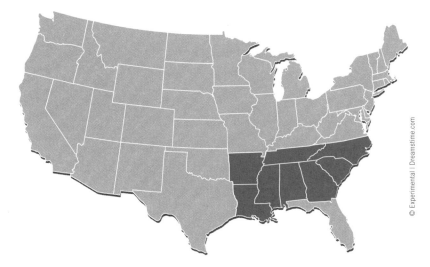

© Experimental | Dreamstime.com

The highest rates of stroke are in the southeastern United States, an area known as the "stroke belt." It includes North Carolina, South Carolina, Georgia, Tennessee, Mississippi, Alabama, Louisiana, and Arkansas.

People who live in stroke belt states have a 20-percent higher risk of dying from stroke than people who live in other states.

Other Risk Factors

Factors that increase risk to a lesser degree include:

▶ Restless legs syndrome. People with restless legs syndrome are twice as likely to have a stroke as people without the disorder. The worse the condition, the greater the risk of stroke.

▶ Heavy drinking. Although alcohol has been shown to have cardiovascular benefits, the key is moderation. Heavy consumption is associated with increased risk of both hemorrhagic and ischemic stroke. Binge drinking may also increase the risk of hemorrhagic stroke.

▶ Psychological distress. Depression and other types of psychological distress increase the risk of stroke. The risk appears to increase in proportion to the extent of the distress. Depression is associated with a two-fold increased risk of a first stroke and 34 percent higher risk of a second stroke. The reason for the link between depression and stroke is unknown.

▶ Inflammation. Tests for two indicators of increased inflammation (high-sensitivity C-reactive protein [hs-CRP] and lipoprotein-associated phospholipase A2 [PLA2]) can improve the ability to predict five-year risk of stroke when added to traditional risk factor assessment. Patients with inflammatory conditions, such as rheumatoid arthritis and lupus, are at increased risk for stroke and should take extra precautions to lower their risk.

PREVENTING STROKES

Stroke is the fifth leading cause of death in the United States. Consider these statistics from the American Stroke Association and the Centers for Disease Control and Prevention:

- Every 40 seconds, someone in this country has a stroke.
- After age 55, the chance of having a stroke doubles with each decade.
- Every year, about 610,000 people have their first stroke, and 185,000 have another stroke.
- Stroke is a leading cause of serious, long-term disability.
- By 2050, the number of strokes is expected to double, with the majority of the increase among patients aged 75 and older and minorities.

> Prevention: Hypertension is the single most important modifiable risk factor for a first or second stroke.

Risk Factors

The encouraging news is that a large percentage of ischemic strokes could be prevented by controlling risk factors. If you have not had a stroke, but have risk factors, you can take steps to prevent a stroke. If you have already had a stroke, and your doctor has advised you on how to minimize your risk of another stroke, following your doctor's advice could lower your risk as much as 65 percent and prolong your life. Moreover, it may improve your quality of life, since many of the same risk factors associated with stroke—particularly high systolic blood pressure, diabetes, and left ventricular hypertrophy—also are associated with cognitive decline.

The Role of Heredity

Some risk factors for stroke are outside of our control. Family history is one of them. The risk of stroke is 50 percent higher in people with a parent or sibling who had a stroke. Heredity is one explanation. However, similar lifestyle habits within families also could be at work. This means that people with a family history of stroke must be extra careful in controlling their risk factors, which we explain on the following pages.

BOX 3-1

Blood Pressure: What's Your Score?

Blood pressure measurements include two numbers, your systolic and diastolic blood pressures, which are expressed in millimeters of mercury (mm Hg). The higher systolic blood pressure is expressed first, followed by the lower diastolic blood pressure. Optimal blood pressure is less than 120/80 mm Hg.

CATEGORY	SYSTOLIC (UPPER NUMBER)	DIASTOLIC (LOWER NUMBER)
Optimal blood pressure	Under 120	Under 80
Prehypertension	120-139	80-89
Stage 1	140-159	90-99
Stage 2	160-179	100-109
Stage 3	180 +	110+

Hypertension

Hypertension is the single most important modifiable risk factor for a first or second stroke. About 77 percent of people who have a first stroke have hypertension, defined as a blood pressure reading higher than 140/90 mmHg. Anyone with a systolic blood pressure of 160 mm Hg or higher and/or a diastolic blood pressure of 95 mm Hg or higher has four times the risk of stroke of someone with normal blood pressure (120/80 mm Hg or less).

Because hypertension rarely produces worrisome symptoms, it has long been called "the silent killer." Most people learn they have hypertension during a routine checkup. If you are prone to frequent headaches, get dizzy more often than you used to, have occasional nosebleeds, and notice that your heart races or beats irregularly from time to time, you may have hypertension. Have your blood pressure checked. It could be normal, or you could have pre-hypertension or hypertension (see Box 3-1, "Blood Pressure: What's Your Score?").

Lowering blood pressure to less than 140/90 mm Hg—130/90 mm Hg after a lacunar stroke (see Box 1-2 on page 11)—has been shown to reduce the risk of a second stroke.

What You Can Do

Take Medication to Lower Blood Pressure

People commonly require two or three drugs to control their blood pressure. There are many to choose from (see Box 3-2, "Drugs That Lower Blood Pressure," on page 39). A few months of trial and error may be needed to find the right drug or combination of drugs and the right doses that work best with the fewest side effects.

- Diuretics work by forcing the kidneys to excrete more salt along with water. Diuretics enhance the effectiveness of other antihypertension drugs. Many diuretics are available in generic form.
- Beta-blockers prevent adrenaline (epinephrine) from constricting the arteries, narrowing the lumen, and raising heart rate and cardiac output.
- Calcium-channel blockers prevent dissolved calcium from entering cells and causing muscles to contract. These medications are useful in preventing the muscle surrounding an artery from constricting it, forcing blood pressure to rise.

- Angiotensin-converting enzyme (ACE) inhibitors prevent the hormone angiotensin from constricting blood vessels and raising blood pressure.
- Angiotensin receptor blockers (ARBs) work differently on angiotensin, but have the same effect.

Nip Hypertension in the Bud

People with blood pressures in the prehypertension range (120-139 mm Hg over 80-89 mm Hg) are at higher risk of developing hypertension and should be screened by a doctor yearly. Self-monitoring with a home blood pressure monitor (available from pharmacies) is also recommended. The doctor may recommend dietary changes, such as lowering salt intake and increasing

BOX 3-2

Drugs That Lower Blood Pressure

Diuretics
- Lasix (furosemide)
- Microzide, Oretic (hydrochlorothiazide)
- Diuril (chlorothiazide)
- Midamor (amiloride)
- Indapamide (Lozol)
- Thaliatone, Hygroton (chlorthalidone)

Beta-Blockers
- Zebeta (bisprolol)
- Corgard (nadolol)
- Inderal (propranolol)
- Tenormin (atenolol)
- Toprol XL, Lopressor (metoprolol)
- Coreg (carvedilol)
- Normodyne, Trandate (labetalol)

Calcium-Channel Blockers
- Cardizem, Tiazac, Dilacor XR (diltiazem)
- Adalat CC, Procardia XL (nifedipine)
- Norvasc (amlodipine)
- Plendil (felodipine)
- Calan, Covera HS, Isoptin, Verelan (verapamil)

ACE Inhibitors
- Capoten (captopril)
- Accupril (quinapril)
- Altace (ramipril)
- Lotensin (benazepril)
- Monopril (fosinopril)
- Vasotec (enalapril)
- Prinivil, Zestril (lisinopril)

ARBs
- Cozaar (losartan)
- Diovan (valsartan)
- Avapro (irbesartan)
- Atacand (candesartan)
- Micardis (telmisartan)

Combinations (partial list)
- Hyzaar (hydrochlorothiazide and losartan)
- Avalide (hydrochlorothiazide and irbesartan)
- Dyazide, Maxzide (hydrochlorothiazide and triamterene)
- Vaseretic (hydrochlorothiazide and enalapril)
- Lexxel (enalapril and felodipine)

BOX 3-3

Top 12 Sources of Sodium

According to the American Heart Association/ American Stroke Association's Heart Disease and Stroke Statistics 2016 update, the top 12 sources of the sodium we consume are:

1. Yeast breads
2. Chicken and chicken mixed dishes
3. Pizza
4. Pasta dishes
5. Cold cuts
6. Condiments
7. Mexican mixed dishes
8. Sausage, franks, bacon, and ribs
9. Cheese
10. Grain-based desserts
11. Soups
12. Beef and beef mixed dishes

exercise. Medication to lower blood pressure may also be prescribed. Your doctor may also suggest:

- Getting at least 3,500 mg of potassium per day from foods such as bananas, dried fruits, skim milk and potatoes.
- Getting at least 1,200 mg of calcium per day from a variety of foods, such as yogurt and skim milk. Low-fat dairy products have been shown to decrease blood pressure.
- Getting enough magnesium from foods such as halibut, dry-roasted almonds and cashews, spinach, whole-grain cereals, black-eyed peas, long-grain brown rice, kidney and pinto beans, avocados, bananas and raisins. Men should aim for 420 mg of magnesium a day; women for 320 mg a day.
- Eating more fiber from whole grains, fruits, vegetables, and nuts—optimally, 25 grams or more. Each 7-gram increase in fiber consumption has been linked to a seven percent decrease in risk of stroke. Increasing fiber may also help lower blood pressure and cholesterol.
- Eating foods containing polyphenols, such as chocolate. Consuming about 30 calories a day worth of dark chocolate—the equivalent of about two Hershey's kisses—may lower blood pressure levels without weight gain or any other negative effects.
- Limiting alcohol consumption.

Get Moving

Aerobic exercise can lower blood pressure while reducing undesirable levels of cholesterol, blood sugar, and stress and increasing energy, feelings of wellbeing, and beneficial HDL cholesterol. It can also help you maintain or lose weight—which is important, because obesity is a risk factor for stroke.

Aerobic exercises are activities that require sustained movement for 30 to 60 minutes, such as walking, running, bicycling, swimming, or dancing. Guidelines released by the American Heart Association/American Stroke Association in 2016 recommend moderate-to-vigorous activity for at least 40 minutes a day on three or four days of the week. The time spent exercising can be spread out over the whole day.

If you've been diagnosed with cardiovascular disease, check with your doctor before beginning any exercise program.

BOX 3-4

Exercise is good for your heart, but you may need to build up your tolerance slowly.

Reduce Salt Consumption

The average American consumes two to three teaspoons of salt per day, but we require only a fraction of that amount. Reducing salt intake to one teaspoon or less may normalize blood pressure if you have mild hypertension and prevent or delay the development of hypertension if you are healthy. One study found that participants who consumed 4,000 or more milligrams of sodium (about two teaspoons of salt) a day were almost three times more likely to suffer a stroke as those who consumed less than 1,500 milligrams of sodium (about ¾ teaspoon of salt) a day. Another study found that stroke risk rises 17 percent with each increase in salt consumption of 500 mg per day.

Most of the sodium we eat comes from processed foods and foods prepared in restaurants (see Box 3-3, "Top 12 Sources of Sodium," on page 40).

In general, sodium should be limited to less than 2,400 milligrams a day (about 1¼ teaspoon of salt). However, people age 51 and older, African-Americans, and those with high blood pressure, diabetes, and chronic kidney disease should keep it under 1,500 milligrams a day.

To lower your sodium intake, read Nutrition Facts labels while shopping, and choose foods with the lowest sodium content. New Nutrition Facts labels will be appearing on food products in the next few years, and will include updated values for sodium and other nutrients based on the latest scientific research. Other changes include making serving sizes and calories easier to read and understand (see Box 3-4, "Old vs. New Nutrition Facts Labels"). Eat plenty of fruits and vegetables (fresh and frozen) and limit processed foods high in sodium. When eating out, request lower sodium meals.

The National Institutes of Health (NIH) developed the Dietary Approaches to Stop Hypertension (DASH) eating plan to help people with systolic blood pressures of 150 mm Hg or more and diastolic blood pressures of 80-95 mm Hg lower their blood pressure. There's a regular DASH eating plan and a

Old vs. New Nutrition Facts Labels

Nutrition Facts
Serving Size 2/3 cup (55g)
Servings Per Container About 8

Amount Per Serving	
Calories 230	Calories from Fat 72

	% Daily Value*
Total Fat 8g	12%
Saturated Fat 1g	5%
Trans Fat 0g	
Cholesterol 0mg	0%
Sodium 160mg	7%
Total Carbohydrate 37g	12%
Dietary Fiber 4g	16%
Sugars 12g	
Protein 3g	

Vitamin A	10%
Vitamin C	8%
Calcium	20%
Iron	45%

* Percent Daily Values are based on a 2,000 calorie diet. Your daily value may be higher or lower depending on your calorie needs.

		Calories:	2,000	2,500
Total Fat	Less than		65g	80g
Sat Fat	Less than		20g	25g
Cholesterol	Less than		300mg	300mg
Sodium	Less than		2,400mg	2,400mg
Total Carbohydrate			300g	375g
Dietary Fiber			25g	30g

▲ **Old Nutrition Label** ▲

Nutrition Facts
8 servings per container
Serving size   2/3 cup (55g)

Amount per serving
Calories   230

	% Daily Value*
Total Fat 8g	12%
Saturated Fat 1g	5%
Trans Fat 0g	
Cholesterol 0mg	0%
Sodium 160mg	7%
Total Carbohydrate 37g	12%
Dietary Fiber 4g	16%
Total Sugars 12g	
Includes 10g Added Sugars	20%
Protein 3g	

Vitamin D 2mcg	10%
Calcium 260mg	20%
Iron 8mg	45%
Potassium 235mg	6%

* The % Daily Value (DV) tells you how much a nutrient in a serving of food contributes to a daily diet. 2,000 calories a day is used for general nutrition advice.

▲ **New Nutrition Label** ▲

fda.gov/Food/GuidanceRegulation/GuidanceDocumentsRegulatoryInformation/LabelingNutrition

BOX 3-5

DASH Facts

The NIH publishes a brochure entitled "Lowering Your Blood Pressure with DASH." To get a copy, you can:

Download from the NIH website
http://bit.ly/2bVypi7

Order by writing
NIH Health Information Center
P.O. Box 30105
Bethesda, MD 20824

low-sodium DASH eating plan. Both are effective, but the low-sodium DASH plan was shown to lower blood pressure to a greater extent (see Box 3-5, "DASH Facts").

Lower Your Cholesterol

If you have an LDL cholesterol level of 100 mg/dL or greater, lowering your LDL with statins can lower your stroke risk, regardless of whether your blood pressure is normal or high. If you have hypertension, lowering your LDL is even more important. Taking medications to bring down both your LDL and blood pressure as far as possible will give you the greatest protection.

Stop Smoking

High blood pressure increases the risk of hemorrhagic stroke, and people with high blood pressure who also smoke have an even higher risk. In a study that enrolled more than 560,000 participants, more than one-third of whom were smokers, researchers found that for every 10 mm Hg increase in systolic blood pressure, smokers had an 81 percent increased risk of hemorrhagic stroke. Smokers with the highest systolic blood pressure readings were nearly 10 times more likely to have a stroke than smokers with the lowest blood pressures.

Atherosclerosis

As you read in Chapter 2, atherosclerosis is a major risk factor for stroke as well as heart attack. The causes of atherosclerosis are well known and include hypertension, smoking, abnormal cholesterol and triglyceride levels, diabetes, obesity, and lack of physical activity. Fortunately, there are many ways to reduce your risk of developing atherosclerosis.

What You Can Do

Stop Using Tobacco

Current smokers have two to four times the risk of ischemic stroke and subarachnoid hemorrhage compared with nonsmokers and those who have quit for more than 10 years.

BOX 3-6

Smoking increases the risk of clotting by raising fibrinogen levels and making platelets stickier. Smoke irritates the lining of the blood vessels and decreases the body's ability to dissolve clots. Smoking is particularly dangerous for young women who suffer from migraine.

The good news is that quitting smoking causes stroke risk to drop fairly quickly. If you are a light-to-moderate smoker, your risk may drop to the same level as a nonsmoker in five years. If you are a heavy smoker, it may take 10 years or more for your risk level to equal that of someone who has never smoked.

There is no question that it's hard to stop smoking, but don't give up. Your chance of success gets better with each try. Most smokers try to quit seven times before they finally succeed. Smoking-cessation aids can be helpful (see Box 3-6, "Tips for Quitting Smoking").

It's also important to avoid exposure to secondhand smoke, which you inhale when you're in the same room as people who are smoking. Secondhand smoke can also increase the risk of stroke.

Although some smokers think that using smokeless tobacco might lower their risk while providing the same gratification as smoking, their reasoning is faulty: A review of studies from two countries found a nearly 50 percent greater risk of fatal stroke among people who had never smoked, but who used smokeless tobacco.

Adjust Your Blood Lipid Levels

Cholesterol and triglycerides are fats (lipids) used to make cell membranes and certain hormones. Triglycerides are the body's main energy-storage molecules and are stored in fat tissue. Although cholesterol and triglycerides are essential for life, having too much increases the risk of developing atherosclerosis. High triglycerides more than double the risk of stroke. For these reasons, cholesterol and triglycerides levels should be kept within normal limits (see Box 3-7, "Cholesterol and Triglyceride Guidelines," on page 44).

Cholesterol and triglyceride levels can be measured with a simple blood test. If they are high, your doctor will recommend lifestyle changes and medications. Achieving a healthy lipid

Tips for Quitting Smoking

- Understand that trying to quit smoking is difficult, so it takes commitment.

- Use more than one stop-smoking aid simultaneously. Studies report increased success among those who use several aids, such as a medication, nicotine patch, and group therapy.

- Don't focus on possible weight gain or try to diet at the same time. The few pounds you might gain are much less of a health risk than smoking.

- Learn to cope with or avoid environments that trigger your urge to smoke.

- Be goal-oriented. Set a definite date to be smoke-free, rather than simply trying to cut back.

- Use mental imagery to imagine yourself as a successful nonsmoker.

- Maximize your chance of success by mobilizing your family, friends and co-workers to support your efforts.

- When you feel a craving for a cigarette, say to yourself, "I can handle it" or "It will go away soon."

- Find a substitute—drink water or milk, eat sugarless candy, start doodling, call a friend on the telephone to help you through it, take a deep breath—anything to distract your mouth and hands.

- If you don't succeed the first time, figure out why you failed and make an extra effort to overcome that reason the next time.

- If you can't seem to do it by yourself, discuss nicotine replacement therapy and smoking cessation programs with your doctor.

BOX 3-7

Cholesterol and Triglyceride Guidelines

Cleveland Clinic cardiologists follow very aggressive guidelines for managing cholesterol levels. Here's how they compare with the National Cholesterol Education Program's (NCEP) guidelines. Although Cleveland Clinic guidelines recommend lower target levels of LDL-cholesterol, total cholesterol and triglycerides, everyone agrees that it is most important for patients to do everything they can to achieve optimal LDL-cholesterol levels. Both Cleveland Clinic and the NCEP advise starting a low-cholesterol, low-fat diet even if you do not have heart disease, have fewer than two heart disease risk factors, and your LDL-cholesterol is less than 160 mg/dL.

All cholesterol values are given in milligrams per deciliter (mg/dL)

		LDL cholesterol [a]	Total cholesterol	HDL cholesterol [b]		Triglycerides
CLEVELAND CLINIC	People without heart disease	<100	<150-175	Men: >40 Women: >50		<150
	People with heart disease	<70	<150	Men: >40 Women: >50		<150
NCEP GUIDELINES	People without heart disease	<160	<200	>40		<150
	People with heart disease	Moderate risk: <130 High risk: <100 Very high risk: < 70	<200	>40		<150

[a] Neither Cleveland Clinic nor the NCEP consider lowering total cholesterol to these levels a therapeutic goal. This is because LDL-cholesterol typically makes up 60 to 70 percent of total serum cholesterol. If LDL-cholesterol targets are met by lifestyle modifications and/or medical therapy, it's almost certain that total cholesterol levels will fall accordingly.

[b] The NCEP has not issued guidelines for raising HDL-cholesterol to a specific goal, although it recognizes low HDL-cholesterol as an independent risk factor for coronary artery disease. NCEP guidelines simply define low and high levels, and encourage adoption of lifestyles and/or drug therapy to raise HDL-cholesterol as part of an overall treatment plan to manage other lipid risk factors, particularly LDL-cholesterol.

profile is especially important if you've already had an ischemic stroke or heart attack, or if you have carotid artery disease or coronary artery disease. An estimated 27 percent of people hospitalized for stroke or transient ischemic attack have LDL levels above those recommended by national guidelines.

Eating a heart-healthy diet can prevent or slow the development of atherosclerosis. Most foods recommended in heart-healthy diets are low in fat and cholesterol and high in nutrients thought to provide additional protection. The American Heart Association recommends getting the right nutrients by eating a variety of foods in moderation. The only nutritional supplement they recommend is omega-3 fatty acids, and only if these cannot be obtained in sufficient amounts from eating fish.

Even if you do everything right, changing your diet may lower your cholesterol by only five to 15 percent. This may be enough for people with borderline high cholesterol. If cholesterol levels are high, medications will be necessary.

BOX 3-8

Take Lipid-Lowering Drugs

Several types of drugs are available to lower total cholesterol, LDL-cholesterol and triglyceride levels. The choice of lipid-lowering drug depends on your individual situation. Your doctor will set goals for you and recommend the drug or drugs with the greatest probability of helping you meet your lipid goals.

Statins

Statins are the first-line cholesterol-lowering drugs, because they are known to reduce fatal and non-fatal ischemic strokes (see Box 3-8, "Statins"). A combined analysis of studies found that every drop of 39 mg/dL in LDL cholesterol achieved with statins lowered the risk of stroke about 21 percent. The effect was seen in people who had never had a stroke, as well as in those at risk of recurrent stroke.

Statins reduce the amount of cholesterol made in the liver. In the process, they lower total cholesterol by 16 to 45 percent and LDL-cholesterol by 20 to 60 percent in two to three weeks. They are effective in men and women of any age and in those who have suffered heart attacks and strokes, as well as those who have not. Statins can also reduce triglyceride levels by up to 25 to 30 percent.

In addition to protecting against a first stroke, statins may help prevent a recurrent stroke. A large study showed that treating stroke patients with statins reduced the risk of a second stroke or a heart attack, even if they were not diagnosed with heart disease. In the study of patients who had suffered a stroke within the previous six months, those taking the statin drug atorvastatin had a 16 percent lower risk for stroke and 35 percent lower risk for a major heart problem compared with those taking a placebo.

Statins might also offer some protection during a stroke by minimizing stroke-related injury. Retrospective analyses of stroke survivors have found that pre-stroke statin users were less likely to experience deterioration in the hospital and more likely to be alive 90 days after their stroke than those who were not taking statins. This may be due to the fact that statin users tend to suffer smaller strokes, which may be the result of an effect of the medication that protects the brain.

Statins

Seven statins are available by prescription:

1. atorvastatin (Lipitor)
2. simvastatin (Zocor)
3. pravastatin (Pravachol)
4. rosuvastatin (Crestor)
5. fluvastatin (Lescol)
6. lovastatin (Mevacor, Altoprev)
7. pitavastatin (Livalo)

The most common side effect of statins is muscle pain. Patients who take statins must undergo periodic blood tests to monitor for liver toxicity and muscle inflammation, although occurrences are rare.

If you are taking statins and suffer a stroke, it's important to continue statin therapy, and not suddenly stop taking the medications, to prevent a rebound effect that can increase the risk of recurrent stroke or death by 300 percent.

In addition to lowering LDL cholesterol, statins reduce levels of C-reactive protein (CRP), a marker of inflammation. CRP may be a better indicator of risk of future cardiovascular events than LDL. Inflammation in the arteries appears to trigger the development of atherosclerosis. Patients with higher levels of CRP are at a higher risk of developing a future heart attack or stroke. One study showed that reducing CRP levels with a statin not only reduced the risk of heart attack, but also reduced the number of ischemic strokes by 51 percent.

Cholesterol Absorption Inhibitors

Ezetimibe (Zetia) is the only drug cholesterol absorption inhibitor available today. It works differently than statins by reducing the absorption of cholesterol from food by more than 50 percent, lowering total cholesterol by about 13 percent, LDL by about 18 percent and triglycerides by about eight percent, and increasing HDL by one percent.

The IMPROVE-IT study, presented in 2014, showed that the combination of ezetimibe and simvastatin (Vytorin) was more effective than simvastatin alone in preventing stroke and heart attack.

Bile Acid Sequestrants

Bile acid sequestrants, such as micronized colestipol (Colestid), colesevelam (WelChol) and cholestyramine (Questran), can also lower cholesterol. These drugs are polymers that bind to bile acids in the small intestine and prevent their reabsorption. Bile acids are made in the liver from cholesterol and stored in the gall bladder for release into the small intestine following a meal. Bile acids are important for the efficient absorption of lipids from food. In the process, most bile acids are absorbed with the lipids and reused. Bile acid sequestrants prevent the reabsorption of bile acids, which forces the liver to make more. This consumes more of the body's cholesterol and reduces total cholesterol, LDL and triglyceride levels, and increases HDL. Bile acid sequestrants are not as effective as statins or ezetimibe. They are also inconvenient, since the dosage involves taking several very large pills a day. Side effects can include constipation and indigestion.

Fibrates

Fibrates (also called fibric acid derivatives) are more effective in lowering triglycerides and raising beneficial HDL than in lowering LDL. Fibrates may raise HDL cholesterol by more than 10 percent and lower triglycerides by almost 30 percent, while reducing LDL and total cholesterol by 20 to 25 percent. Therefore, fibrates are often prescribed in addition to statins for patients with very high cholesterol levels or to patients who cannot tolerate statins. Patients who take fibrates require periodic liver function tests to monitor for liver injury and gallstone formation.

Niacin

Niacin is in the B vitamin family, which also includes thiamine and riboflavin. When taken with meals three times a day in rather large doses (two to six grams a day), niacin can raise HDL by 20 to 25 percent, but it is not as effective as fibrates in lowering triglycerides. At therapeutic doses, niacin almost always causes flushing and itching, which many patients find difficult or impossible to tolerate. Controlled- or extended-release formulations such as Niaspan or Slo-Niacin have fewer side effects. If you have very low HDL, Niaspan in combination with a statin is preferred over a fibrate. However, the combination slightly increases the risk of side effects.

Obesity

According to the American Heart Association, 69 percent of U.S. adults are overweight or obese, and the percentage is steadily rising. This is a serious problem, because obesity is a risk factor for every cardiovascular disease, including stroke. It is also a risk factor for death from stroke. In fact, the more overweight you are, the greater your risk of stroke. One study found the risk of ischemic stroke was 22 percent higher among people who were overweight and 64 percent higher among those who were obese, compared with people of normal weight.

One way to determine if you are overweight or obese is to calculate your body mass index (see Box 3-9, "What's Your Body Mass Index?"). If you are in the overweight or obese category, you should seriously consider changing how you eat and starting to exercise. If you are a man and 100 pounds over your ideal weight, or a woman carrying an extra 80 pounds, you are considered morbidly obese. This means your obesity is highly likely to cause medical problems. Your doctors may prescribe a weight-loss drug for you or recommend bariatric surgery.

What You Can Do

Eat Right

The key to losing weight is to improve your food choices and eating habits (see Box 3-10, "Keys to a Weight-Loss Diet," on page 49). The American Heart Association and National Cholesterol Education Program recommend a diet in which only

BOX 3-9

What's Your Body Mass Index?

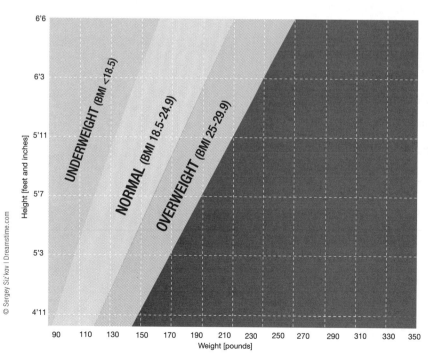

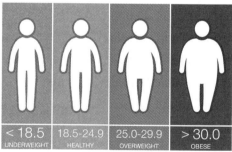

Body mass index (BMI) is one method used to determine obesity. You can estimate your BMI by finding your weight and height in the chart on the left, or you can use easy online BMI calculators.

A BMI of over 25 is considered overweight, and over 30 is obese.

© Sergey Siz'kov | Dreamstime.com

BOX 3-10

eight to 10 percent of calories come from saturated fats, 10 percent or less from polyunsaturated fats, and 15 percent or less from monounsaturated fats. Experts agree that the most successful weight-loss programs involve making changes that you can stick with over time. Losing a pound or two each week is a reasonable goal.

Weight-loss drugs are an option, but many have serious side effects. Alli (orlistat) is half the strength of its prescription predecessor, Xenical. Alli works by blocking the absorption of fat in the gastrointestinal tract. As a result, it has some of the same side effects that plagued Xenical, namely gas, oily discharge, inability to control bowel movements, oily or fatty stools, and oily spotting. Yet people who take Alli, follow a low-fat diet, and exercise can lose 50 percent more weight than with diet and exercise alone.

Vitamins and Nutrients

In addition to eating healthier foods and preparing them in a healthy way, eat a nutritionally rich diet including foods from all food groups. This way, you will be sure to get the full complement of vitamins you need to stay healthy.

Getting adequate amounts of vitamin D is important, since brain damage can be greater after a stroke in patients with low vitamin D levels. Moreover, those with low vitamin D levels were less likely to be functionally independent three months post-stroke.

The primary sources of vitamin D are fatty fish, egg yolks, fortified milk and cereals, and sunlight. Unacceptably low vitamin D levels can be raised with supplements of 1,000 to 2,000 international units (IU) per day, then maintained with doses of 200 to 600 IU daily.

It also appears to be important to incorporate foods with vitamin B-6 and folate in the diet. Studies have found that folate and vitamin B-6 protects women from fatal stroke and heart attack and men from heart failure death. The researchers believe these two vitamins may protect against cardiovascular disease by lowering levels of homocysteine. Excess amounts of this amino acid are known to damage the linings of the arteries and promote the formation of blood clots.

Keys to a Weight-Loss Diet

- Eat a lot of fruits and vegetables.
- Steam or grill meats instead of frying them. As an alternative, lightly oil and bread meats and bake them for a healthier "oven-fried" taste.
- Replace simple carbohydrates, such as white bread, with complex carbohydrates, such as whole grain breads and cereals and brown rice.
- Reduce your portion sizes.
- If you need help losing weight, make an appointment with a registered dietitian or join a group program such as Weight Watchers.

BOX 3-11

Conditions of Metabolic Syndrome

A person with metabolic syndrome has three or more of the following conditions:

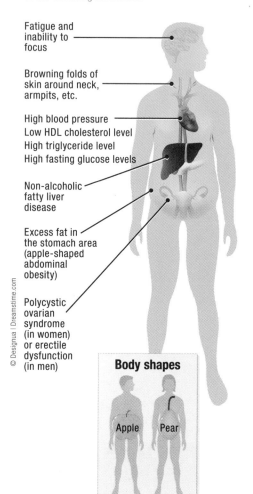

Fatigue and inability to focus

Browning folds of skin around neck, armpits, etc.

High blood pressure
Low HDL cholesterol level
High triglyceride level
High fasting glucose levels

Non-alcoholic fatty liver disease

Excess fat in the stomach area (apple-shaped abdominal obesity)

Polycystic ovarian syndrome (in women) or erectile dysfunction (in men)

Body shapes

Apple   Pear

© Designua | Dreamstime.com

Be Physically Active

Regular physical activity significantly reduces your risk of any cardiovascular disease, including stroke. One study found that people who engaged in physical activity less than four times per week had a 20 percent greater risk of stroke than those who exercised four or more times per week. This effect may be largely due to the effect of exercise on reducing other risk factors, such as obesity and diabetes.

Research also suggests moderate-to-intense physical activity may protect the brain from so-called "silent strokes." These strokes do not produce the normal stroke symptoms (see Box 1-5 on page 14), but rather contribute to mental decline and dementia, and increase the risk of a subsequent stroke.

To help your heart and brain stay healthy, try to perform some physical activity for at least 30 minutes every day. If you need to lose weight, aim for one hour a day. The time can be broken up into shorter segments, such as walks or bike rides in the morning and again after dinner. Keep in mind that the regularity of physical activity is more important than the intensity of the workout. Ordinary tasks like yard work and housecleaning also count as physical activity.

The key to getting in shape is to find an activity that you like to do. The more physical activity you do, the more fit you'll become, and improved fitness is associated with better cardiovascular health.

If you have had a stroke, have risk factors for cardiovascular disease, or are elderly or sedentary, ask your doctor for advice about what kind of exercise and what intensity level is safe for you. Your doctor may want to make sure your blood pressure and cholesterol are under control before you begin.

Metabolic Syndrome

The term "metabolic syndrome" is used to define a cluster of risk factors for cardiovascular disease (see Box 3-11, "Conditions of Metabolic Syndrome"). The presence of metabolic syndrome in people with atherosclerosis increases the risk for ischemic stroke or TIA.

What You Can Do

Metabolic syndrome is treated by addressing the individual components—losing weight, lowering cholesterol levels and blood pressure, and correcting blood sugar levels.

Diabetes Mellitus

Diabetes increases the risk of stroke two to eight times, and also increases the risk of heart disease and peripheral arterial disease. Women with diabetes have a greater risk of stroke than men with diabetes (see Box 3-12, "The Mars and Venus of Stroke"). The longer a person has diabetes, the higher the risk for stroke.

As shown in Box 3-13, "Type-2 Diabetes: A Disorder of Sugar Metabolism," diabetes is primarily a disorder of sugar metabolism. There are two types: Type 1 diabetes is also called insulin-dependent diabetes mellitus. It is an autoimmune disease in which the immune system attacks the cells in the pancreas that make insulin. As a result, the pancreas is unable to make enough insulin or cannot make it at all.

Ninety percent of the 18 million Americans who have diabetes

BOX 3-12

The Mars and Venus of Stroke

Researchers have started uncovering significant biological and physiological differences between men and women. Sex-based biology, also known as gender-specific medicine, has all but revolutionized the way that doctors view—and treat—women and men. Stroke is no exception.

Findings on the gender differences in stroke include:

- Each year, about 55,000 more women than men have a stroke.
- On average, women are about four years older than men at the time of their stroke.
- Women account for 60 percent of stroke deaths.
- Men with acute ischemic stroke are more likely to benefit from tPA than women.
- Women with female relatives who had an ischemic stroke are at higher risk of having a stroke than men with affected relatives.
- Women with diabetes are less likely than men with diabetes to survive a stroke.

BOX 3-13

Type 2 Diabetes: A Disorder of Sugar Metabolism

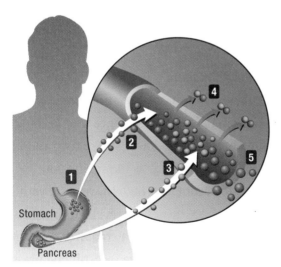

1. Stomach converts food to glucose.

2. Glucose enters the bloodstream.

3. Pancreas produces sufficient insulin but it is resistant to effective use.

4. Glucose unable to enter to the body effectively.

5. Blood glucose levels increase.

© Rob3000 | Dreamstime.com

have type 2 diabetes. For reasons that are not completely understood, muscle and fat cells become unable to respond to insulin, no matter how much the pancreas makes. As a result, blood sugar levels rise. This defect is called insulin resistance. Type 2 diabetes has traditionally occurred after the age of 40, hence it is also called "adult-onset" diabetes. However, a growing number of young people and children are being diagnosed with the disease due to obesity. Type 2 diabetes is closely linked to obesity, high blood pressure and high cholesterol.

What You Can Do

Control Your Blood Sugar

For many reasons, including lowering the risk of stroke, people with diabetes need to take steps to control their blood sugar levels with diet, exercise, and medications. People with type 1 diabetes require daily insulin injections. Most people with type 2 diabetes will take oral glucose-lowering drugs called "insulin-sensitizing agents," the most common being metformin (Glucophage). It enhances the insulin sensitivity of the cells, enabling them to remove sugar from the bloodstream with less insulin. If diet, exercise, and metformin do not adequately lower blood sugar levels, there are several other types of drugs that your doctor may prescribe. Some people with type 2 diabetes need to take insulin to manage their blood sugar levels.

Control Your Blood Pressure

If you have diabetes, your blood pressure should be less than 140/90 mm Hg. There is strong evidence that keeping tight control of blood pressure can lower stroke risk. You may try lifestyle modifications, such as improving your diet and exercising more, to accomplish this. However, if your blood pressure does not fall to the desired level within a few months, medications will be necessary. It may require more than one anti-hypertension drug to reach the target blood pressure.

Take a Statin and, Maybe, Aspirin

Your doctor may recommend that you take a statin. Studies suggest that statins decrease the risk of a first stroke in patients with diabetes. Your doctor may also recommend daily aspirin.

However, the value of aspirin for preventing a first stroke in patients with diabetes and a low risk for cardiovascular disease is unclear (see Box 3-14, "Aspirin, Statins Reduce Stroke Risk in People With Diabetes").

Atrial Fibrillation

Atrial fibrillation is a powerful risk factor for stroke. People with atrial fibrillation—women in particular—are five times more likely to have a stroke than people without this arrhythmia. Moreover, if you have a stroke caused by atrial fibrillation, you are more than twice as likely to be disabled or bedridden. Because atrial fibrillation is often asymptomatic, it may be the underlying cause of stroke in up to 23 percent of patients in whom the cause of stroke is not identified.

If you have been diagnosed with or suspected to have atrial fibrillation, your doctor may order one or more of the tests listed on page 54.

BOX 3-14

Aspirin, Statins Reduce Stroke Risk in People With Diabetes

The American Diabetes Association makes the following recommendations for aspirin and statin therapy in people with diabetes:

Low-Dose Aspirin Recommended

A low dose (75-162 mg/day) is recommended for patients with type 2 diabetes who have had a heart attack, vascular bypass procedure, stroke or transient ischemic attack, peripheral vascular disease, claudication and/or angina. For patients who have an aspirin allergy, the drug clopidogrel may be used instead of aspirin.

Low-Dose Aspirin Considered

Aspirin at a low dose (75-162 mg/day) may be considered for patients with type 1 or type 2 diabetes who have not had vascular disease, but are at increased risk for cardiovascular disease. This includes most men over 50 years of age, and women over 60 who have at least one additional major risk factor, such as family history of cardiovascular disease, high blood pressure, smoking, high cholesterol, or albumin in their urine (albuminuria).

Aspirin Not Recommended

Daily aspirin is not recommended for patients with diabetes who have not had vascular disease and are at low risk for cardiovascular disease. This includes men under age 50, and women under age 60 with no major additional risk factors, such as family history of cardiovascular disease, high blood pressure, smoking, high cholesterol, or albumin in their urine (albuminuria).

Statin Therapy is Recommended for:

Patients with diabetes and coronary artery disease or other cardiovascular disease, regardless of baseline LDL-cholesterol levels. The goal is an LDL-cholesterol level of less than 70 mg/dL, which will require intensive lipid-lowering therapy.

- Patients over age 40 who do not have cardiovascular disease but have one or more other risk factors for cardiovascular disease. The goal for these patients is an LDL-cholesterol level less than 100 mg/dL.

- Diabetic patients who are under age 40 and do not have cardiovascular disease, statin therapy is recommended if LDL cholesterol remains over 100 mg/dL or the person has several risk factors for cardiovascular disease.

BOX 3-15

How an ECG is Read

An electrocardiogram (ECG) provides a snapshot of the electrical impulses that make the heart beat.

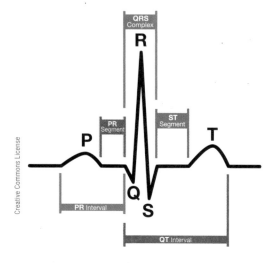

The first recorded electrical oscillation is called the P wave, and it represents the impulse from the sinoatrial node that stimulates atrial contraction.

A series of three waves—Q, R and S—stimulates ventricular contraction.

The T wave represents the relaxation of the ventricular muscle.

A normal heart rate is 60-100 beats per minute. The duration of the ECG trace is about two-thirds of a second, and it becomes even shorter when the heart beats faster during exercise.

ECG is sometimes abbreviated EKG from the German elektrokardiogramm.

ECG

An ECG (sometimes referred to as an EKG) is a noninvasive test that reveals the electrical activity of the heart and can confirm the diagnosis of atrial fibrillation (see Box 3-15, "How an ECG is Read").

Holter Monitor

A 24-hour ambulatory heart-monitoring device called a Holter monitor can help determine whether your atrial fibrillation is persistent or intermittent, and evaluate the effectiveness of prescribed treatments.

Prolonged Home Telemetry

When there is no clear reason for TIA or stroke, home telemetry lasting 30 days or longer may be performed to look for unrecognized atrial fibrillation. The monitors used for this test send signals via satellite to a recording center, which notifies the physician when an arrhythmia is detected.

Echocardiogram

This noninvasive test uses sound waves to reveal the structure and function of the beating heart. A probe slides across the chest, sending and receiving high-frequency ultrasound waves that are bounced off the heart, enabling the doctor to see the heart from different angles. A recording device translates the sound waves into images that clearly reveal any abnormalities in the heart and show how well it pumps. Echocardiograms can show leaky or narrowed heart valves, and an enlarged left atrium, which may suggest atrial fibrillation, as well as holes between the chambers (septal defects or fistulas). All of these increase the risk of stroke.

Transesophageal Echocardiogram (TEE)

This works the same way as a regular echocardiogram to image your heart, but in this test, the tiny sound transducer is located on the end of a long, thin, flexible tube, which is threaded down your esophagus to the level of your heart. Placing the transducer next to the heart enables it to capture greater detail. TEE can reveal the presence of a blood clot in the left atrium with the potential to cause a stroke. This test also provides the best image of the aortic arch, a potential source of embolic stroke.

What You Can Do

Treat Atrial Fibrillation

Your doctor will help you determine the best medical therapy be calculating your risk of stroke, as well as the risk of major bleeding complications from treatment. If you have atrial fibrillation and are a women older than 65 or have another medical condition such as hypertension, heart failure, diabetes, vascular disease, or a history of stroke, you are likely to be prescribed an oral anticoagulant such as warfarin (Coumadin), dabigatran (Pradaxa), rivaroxaban (Xarelto), apixaban (Eliquis), or edoxaban (Savaysa) unless the risk of major bleeding complications is greater than your stroke risk (see Box 3-16, "Reversal Agents Make Novel Blood Thinners Safer"). Patients who do not meet these criteria may be prescribed aspirin alone.

Drugs to slow the heart rate and normalize its rhythm may also be prescribed. A beta-blocker or calcium channel blocker may be used to slow down the accelerated ventricular heart rate that often accompanies atrial fibrillation.

If medical therapy does not stop atrial fibrillation, or antithrombotic therapy is too risky, closing off the atrial appendage where most clots develop may be recommended. This catheter-based treatment is discussed in Chapter 4.

Obstructive Sleep Apnea

As discussed in the last chapter, obstructive sleep apnea (OSA) is an independent risk factor for stroke. Studies have shown that patients with OSA are twice as likely to die following a stroke than patients without OSA. Researchers think that cerebral blood flow and blood pressure increase during the apnea episodes when patients stop breathing, then rapidly drop when the apnea ends (see Box 3-17, "The Anatomy of Obstructive Sleep Apnea"). This indicates the brain fails to receive sufficient oxygen during apnea episodes. Recent guidelines recommend that a sleep study be considered in patients following a TIA or ischemic stroke.

BOX 3-17

The Anatomy of Obstructive Sleep Apnea

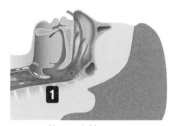 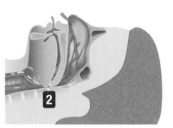

Normal Airway   **Obstructive Sleep Apnea**

© Alila07 | Dreamstime.com

In a normal airway, breathing is free and unobstructed during sleep. In someone with obstructive sleep apnea (OSA), the tissues at the back of the mouth and throat collapse, narrowing or blocking the airway, causing loud snoring and frequent interruptions in breathing (apneas). In severe cases of OSA, apneas may occur hundreds of times a night.

The top-left illustration shows normal breathing and an unobstructed airway (1).

The top-right illustration shows the side view of the upper airway with an obstruction in the back of the throat preventing airflow (2).

BOX 3-18

CPAP Masks

CPAP masks are available in a variety of styles—
see below for some of the examples. Try on several
to find the one that is most comfortable for you.

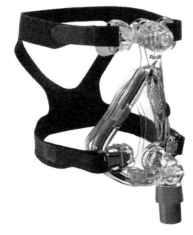

Full Face Mask

Mirage Quattro, Resmed

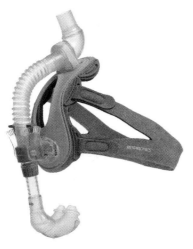

Nasal Mask

ComfortLife 2, Phillips Respironics

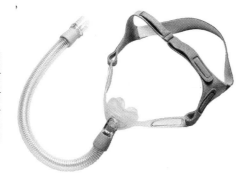

Nasal Pillows

Nuance Pro, Phillips Respironics

What You Can Do

OSA is a treatable condition. If you have OSA, you should avoid alcohol and sedatives before bed. If you are overweight, losing weight may help, as can sleeping on your side. However, these changes may not be enough.

Your doctor may prescribe a device called a continuous positive airway pressure (CPAP) machine. With CPAP, you will wear a mask over your mouth and nose at night, and the machine will blow enough air into them to keep your airway open (see Box 3-18, "CPAP Masks"). Most patients are able to adjust to the machine and find they get more restful sleep with CPAP, in addition to lowering their risk of heart attack and stroke.

Sometimes, surgery is recommended to remove the tonsils or excess tissue in the back of the throat. In some cases of milder apnea, the doctor may prescribe a retainer-like device that is worn at night to reposition the jaw.

What's Next?

If you have any risk factors for stroke, you would be wise to do whatever you can to reduce or eliminate them. Ask your doctor to periodically reassess your condition to determine if your risk of stroke has changed. Keep taking your medications as prescribed.

If your risk of stroke remains high, and your doctor discovers a condition that can be treated with an interventional procedure or surgery, you may want to discuss the risks and benefits. Many of these procedures have been proven to prolong lives and preserve quality of life.

PROCEDURES TO PREVENT STROKE

If your disease has progressed so far that medical therapy is no longer sufficient, you may need an interventional procedure or surgery to prevent a fatal or disabling stroke.

Interventional procedures have many advantages. They are minimally invasive, so recovery is faster and less time in the hospital is required than for traditional surgery. Some procedures can be performed without general anesthesia. Patients are usually able to return to normal activities within a very short period of time. As better devices and techniques have been developed, interventional procedures are gradually replacing surgery. Nevertheless, surgery is still sometimes necessary.

Interventional and surgical procedures for stroke prevention and treatment can be broadly divided into three categories:

1. Those that widen or reopen the interior diameter of arteries in the brain or leading to the brain that contain dangerously large atherosclerotic plaques. These procedures are designed to restore blood flow to the brain and lower the risk of blood clots.

2. Those that treat the heart to reduce the risk of a blood clot that can travel to the brain and cause a stroke.

3. Those that correct structural defects in arteries, making them less prone to rupturing or bursting.

Your doctor will carefully assess your condition and decide whether or not you are eligible for a particular procedure and, if so, whether the risk of stroke outweighs the risk of the procedure.

Procedures to Reopen Arteries

An ischemic stroke occurs when plaque blocks the carotid arteries or ruptures, preventing blood from reaching the brain. Two types of procedures are used to reopen blocked carotid arteries and reduce the risk of stroke. The right choice for you depends on many factors, including your age and the need for cardiac bypass surgery (see Box 4-1, "Combining Heart and Brain Revascularization Procedures").

BOX 4-1

Combining Heart and Brain Revascularization Procedures

Because the disease that causes ischemic strokes—atherosclerosis—can affect other arteries and the organs they serve, many people at risk for stroke are also at risk for heart attack, and vice versa. Patients who require coronary artery bypass surgery (CABG) may also have significant blockages in their carotid arteries and require stroke-prevention surgery. The optimal strategy and timing for treating both problems has been unknown.

Cleveland Clinic heart surgeons explored the outcomes of different revascularization protocols in 350 patients undergoing CABG: 1) carotid endarterectomy, followed by CABG an average of two weeks later, 2) simultaneous carotid endarterecomy and CABG under a single anesthesia, and 3) carotid artery stenting, followed by CABG an average of 47 days later. The patients were then followed for up to 12 years.

As reported in 2013, the most strokes in the first year occurred in the combined endarterectomy-CABG group. Over the long term, those who underwent stenting first, followed by CABG, fared the best.

Results of Endarterectomy and Stenting Equally Good

Two studies presented at the International Stroke Conference in February 2016 reassured physicians that both carotid endarterectomy and stenting produce comparable results that are very good.

The Asymptomatic Carotid Trial 1 (ACT 1) examined both procedures in asymptomatic patients with severe carotid stenosis. They found stenting and endarterectomy to have similar rates of stroke, heart attack, and death within 30 days of the procedure, as well as stroke on the same side as the procedure between 31 days and one year. Rates of death and stroke at five years were also similar.

The Carotid Revascularization Endarterectomy versus Stenting Trial (CREST) found the risk of combined complications—stroke, heart attack, and death—to be very low at less than 0.7 percent per year. The rate of a second stroke on the same side of the body at 10 years after the procedure was the same for both groups. However, the risk of post-procedure stroke was slightly higher with stenting—6.9 percent, compared with 5.6 percent for endarterectomy. These rates are comparable to those in the general population.

New England Journal of Medicine, February 17, 2016

Endarterectomy Reduces Risk of Procedure-Related Stroke in Older, Symptomatic Patients

A review of four randomized, controlled clinical trials comparing carotid endarterectomy with carotid stenting in older, symptomatic patients revealed better outcomes with endarterectomy. Researchers wondered what impact age had on outcomes, and took a closer look at these studies. They divided symptomatic participants into five-year age groups, and assessed rates of stroke or death in the period between enrollment and randomization and 120 days after the procedure. They also looked at rates of recurrent stroke on the same side over the long term. Their findings revealed a higher rate of stroke and death in patients aged 70 and older who underwent carotid stenting, but no increased risk with endarterectomy. Age had no effect on long-term risk with either procedure.

Lancet, March 26, 2016

Carotid endarterectomy has been performed for more than 50 years; stenting is a newer procedure. Initially, the results of endarterectomy were better than those of stenting. But as doctors have gained experience with stenting, and the procedure has been performed on thousands of patients, the short- and long-term results of both procedures have become comparable (see Box 4-2, "Results of Endarterectomy and Stenting Equally Good"). Still, many physicians have a preference for one technique over the other, and there's some evidence that endarterectomy may be a better choice for older patients with symptomatic disease (see Box 4-3, "Endarterectomy Reduces Risk of Procedure-Related Stroke in Older, Symptomatic Patients").

Carotid Endarterectomy

Plaques often form where the common carotid artery divides into the internal and external carotid arteries, a junction called a bifurcation (see Box 4-4, "Carotid Endarterectomy," on page 59). A surgical procedure called carotid endarterectomy is used to remove plaques located at or near the bifurcation that have enlarged to the point they may cause a stroke.

With the identification of modifiable risk factors for stroke and better medical treatments to lower stroke risk in patients without stroke symptoms, the benefit of carotid endarterectomy or stenting has become controversial. Clinical trials now underway will eventually determine which approach is optimal.

Carotid endarterectomy or stenting is routinely offered to all patients with symptomatic carotid artery disease and a blockage of 70 percent or greater—provided they have no other medical problems significant enough to preclude a good outcome, and provided the surgeon's or interventionalist's complication rate is less than six percent. In these patients, the procedure can reduce the risk of stroke by 50 percent over a five-year period.

Symptomatic patients with a 50 to 69 percent blockage are selected to undergo the procedure based on the severity of their symptoms, the presence of other risk factors for stroke, and their medical suitability. For these patients, carotid endarterectomy results in a significant reduction in risk.

How Endarterctomy is Done

Carotid endarterectomy is a surgical procedure requiring anesthesia. Nevertheless, it is relatively simple. Because the carotid arteries lie fairly close to the skin, it is not necessary to cut the muscles of the neck to expose the artery; they are simply moved out of the way.

The surgeon makes a small incision in the neck just below the jaw and separates the neck muscles to expose the diseased carotid artery. Blood flow through the carotid artery is diverted around the blockage with a tube (shunt). A lengthwise incision in the carotid artery is made to expose the blockage. The plaque is carefully removed, and the incision in the artery is sewn shut.

If the plaque has weakened the carotid artery wall, the diseased area is patched and strengthened with a piece of a vein from the leg. The shunt is removed, and the holes where it was inserted are sewn closed, allowing normal blood flow through the carotid artery. Finally, the skin incision is neatly closed.

The entire procedure typically takes less than two hours. Patients remain overnight in the hospital and are discharged the following day. They are usually able to resume their normal activities in a few days. A stiff, achy neck can be relieved by over-the-counter pain medications.

Carotid Stenting

Carotid stenting is another option. In this procedure, a catheter tipped with an inflatable balloon is threaded through the arteries to the site of the plaque. The balloon is inflated, which presses the plaque into the artery wall and out of the way. A small, cylindrical cage called a stent is then inserted in the area of the plaque to provide structural support to the artery and prevent the plaque from recoiling or rebounding. Once the stent is in its intended location, it automatically expands (see Box 4-5, "Stent Deployment"). Cerebrovascular stents are made of nitinol, a nickel alloy that is flexible enough to accommodate the motion of head and neck turning. After the stent is in place, it is dilated with the balloon to the size of the carotid artery to create the maximum vessel diameter.

BOX 4-4

Carotid Endarterectomy

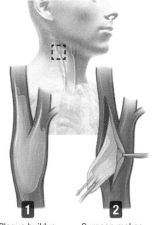

© Eraxion | Dreamstime.com; National Institute of Health

1 Plaque buildup in carotid artery reduces blood flow.

2 Surgeon makes incision in artery wall and removes plaque.

3 The incision is repaired and normal blood flow is restored.

Plaque buildup at the junction (bifurcation) where the carotid artery divides into the external and internal carotid arteries can lead to stroke if the blocked arteries are not reopened in time.

An endarterectomy involves opening the artery and removing the plaque causing the blockage.

BOX 4-5

Stent Deployment

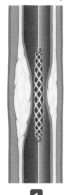 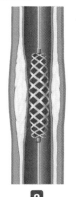 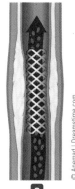

© Anemad | Dreamstime.com

1 A collapsed stent on a balloon catheter is threaded to the area of the plaque.

2 The balloon is inflated, expanding the stent and pressing it against the plaque. This causes a slight bulge in the artery. The balloon catheter is then deflated and removed.

3 The stent is in place.

Before stenting begins, an embolus-protection device may be deployed downstream from the plaque. These devices are tiny collapsible nets that resemble an umbrella or sieve with holes large enough for blood cells to pass through and small enough to trap anything larger, including pieces of plaque. After the stent has been expanded, the embolus-protection device is collapsed and withdrawn along with any plaque debris it may have captured.

Carotid stenting is FDA-approved for all patients with clogged carotid arteries who are at risk for stroke.

How Stenting is Done

The doctor numbs the groin or arm with local anesthetic and makes a small incision in the artery. A short tube called a sheath is inserted in this incision.

A thin, flexible guide wire tipped by an embolus-protection device is inserted through the sheath and threaded past the plaque in the carotid artery. A catheter with a stent is then inserted through the sheath, threaded into the carotid artery, and positioned across the plaque. A contrast agent is injected periodically to allow the doctor to visualize blood flow through the carotid artery on the video X-ray. A balloon catheter is inserted to expand the stent. Finally, the embolus-protection device is folded and withdrawn, along with the guide wire.

In the recovery area, the sheath is withdrawn, and pressure is applied to the puncture site, or a special wound-closure device or sealant is used to prevent bleeding.

The entire procedure usually takes about two hours. The patient may have to lie completely still for several hours to prevent the puncture site from opening and bleeding, but should be able to go home the day after the procedure. It is necessary to take clopidogrel (Plavix) and aspirin daily for at least one month after the procedure.

Intracranial Stenting

Intracranial atherosclerosis accounts for 10 to 15 percent of ischemic strokes in the United States, and patients who have one stroke of this type are at high risk of having another. Patients with blockages greater than 50 percent with a recent stroke

BOX 4-6

or TIA have an 11 percent risk of recurrent stroke within a year, even with antithrombotic therapy. The risk is higher—23 percent—for patients with blockages of 70 percent or more.

The Stenting and Aggressive Medical Management for Preventing Recurrent Stroke in Intracranial Stenosis (SAMMPRIS) trial compared medical management with stenting plus best medical management in nearly 800 patients. The rate of stroke was found to be higher in the stented group than in the medical treatment-only group. Aggressive medical therapy directed at known risk factors for stroke resulted in a lower-than- expected risk of future stroke, reinforcing the need to control risk factors, such as high blood pressure, high cholesterol, diabetes, obesity, and the others described in Chapter 3. The SAMMPRIS investigators concluded that the only patients who may benefit from stenting are those with arteries that are 70 to 90 percent blocked, who have had two or more strokes despite optimal medical treatment, and whose last stroke occurred more than seven days earlier.

Procedures to Reduce the Risk of Blood Clots

Atrial fibrillation (see page 27) is a common cause of stroke, primarily from clots that form in the atrial appendage of the heart. When patients with atrial fibrillation cannot take oral anticoagulants, a number of different methods to seal off (occlude) this pocket in the heart are available. Several surgical techniques have been developed, but they actually increase the risk of clot formation. Other, less-invasive procedures are more commonly used.

Additionally, a procedure called ablation can often stop atrial fibrillation from occurring by eliminating cells on the heart's surface that are sending the wrong electrical signals.

Atrial Appendage Occlusion

Two devices have been created to prevent blood from entering the atrial appendage. They work in different ways. The Watchman device plugs the entrance to the sac, while the Lariat chokes it off from the circulation. Neither device prevents stroke entirely, and some physicians continue to prefer anti-clotting medications for the prevention of atrial fibrillation (see Box 4-6, "Watchman vs Lariat vs Drugs").

Watchman vs Lariat vs Drugs

Oral anticoagulants are highly effective in preventing stroke caused by atrial fibrillation. And with several patient-friendly alternatives to warfarin (Coumadin) now available, doctors are taking a hard look at atrial appendage occluders. These devices are designed to close off the left atrial appendage, a small pouch connected to the left atrium that can sometimes be the source of clot formation.

The Watchman was approved in March 2015 for treating nonvalvular atrial fibrillation following the results of the PREVAIL and PROTECT AF trials. Both compared the device to warfarin therapy, and both found the Watchman to be a safe and effective alternative to warfarin. However, neither found the device to be superior to the medication.

Technically, the Lariat device should eliminate the need for anticoagulants, because the lasso isolates the atrial appendage from the atrium proper. However, the device can leak, and there have been several reports of left atrial clots. No clinical trial has been done comparing the Lariat to long-term anticoagulation.

For these reasons, most doctors prefer anticoagulation for patients at low risk for bleeding. For those who cannot tolerate anticoagulants, atrial appendage occlusion may be an acceptable option.

Ablation

In ablation, high-frequency electrical impulses are sent through a catheter to destroy (ablate) the abnormal cells causing an arrhythmia. Cardiologists call these cells "hot spots."

In order to locate the cells, a cardiologist who specializes in arrhythmias (electrophysiologist) will perform an electrophysiology (EP) study. A special diagnostic catheter is inserted into a vein in the leg or neck and advanced into the right atrium, right ventricle, and location near the Bundle of His (a band of fibers that conducts electrical signals). Electrodes in the catheter transmit information about the heart's electrical activity. The electrophysiologist uses this information to evaluate the heart's electrical system and pinpoint the source of the arrhythmia. Programmed electrical stimulation is then used to deliver electrical signals through the catheter to increase the heart rate. If an arrhythmia occurs, the electrophysiologist will administer anti-arrhythmic medication through an intravenous catheter and evaluate its ability to stop the arrhythmia. Based on the findings of the EP study, the doctor may decide to conduct an ablation procedure or implant a pacemaker or implantable cardioverter-defibrillator (ICD, a small battery-powered electrical impulse generator).

Types of Ablation

The most common type of ablation employs high-energy radio waves to destroy the cells. Other types of catheter ablations freeze the hot spots (cryotherapy) or vaporize the tissue with lasers. The procedure may take several hours.

If the hot spots cannot be pinpointed, the atrioventricular (AV) node may be ablated as a last resort. The AV node receives the electrical signal from the atrium and delays it before sending it on to the ventricles. Once the AV node has been ablated, a pacemaker must be implanted to provide rhythm cues for the ventricles.

After ablation, patients must continue to take anti-clotting medications.

Maze Surgery

All interventional techniques used to treat atrial fibrillation can also be done surgically. The surgical approach is often used in patients with atrial fibrillation who also need open-heart surgery for valve repair, coronary artery bypass, or other reasons. It is not normally done only for stroke prevention. The maze procedure, which was developed at Cleveland Clinic, requires a series of precise incisions to be made in the right and left atria to interrupt the conduction of abnormal impulses and direct sinus impulses to travel to the AV node as they should.

Closing a Patent Foramen Ovale (PFO)

In Chapter 2, we explained how a hole between the left and right atria might fail to close at birth. This allows blood to flow from the right atrium into the left atrium when the pressure in the right atrium is higher. When a blood clot makes its way into the heart, it can pass through the PFO and be pumped to the brain, where it causes an ischemic stroke.

Although PFOs may occur in 20 to 25 percent of the general population, most cause no symptoms, so patients are unaware they have one. However, a PFO is often discovered during the evaluation of a TIA/stroke patient, who appears to have no other explanation for the event. Although a PFO can be closed surgically or with an interventional device, closing the hole with one of these interventional techniques does not appear to be significantly better than medication at reducing the risk of a second stroke.

Procedures to Prevent Intracerebral Hemorrhage

Intracerebral hemorrhages occur in some of the smallest arteries of the brain. Most are too small to access with today's catheters or are located too deep within the brain for surgical repair. Consequently, preventing hypertension-related intracerebral hemorrhages by controlling blood pressure control is advised.

Aneurysms (bulging areas of an artery) found on the larger arteries that branch off the internal carotid, basilar, and vertebral arteries can be treated with interventional procedures or surgery. Arteriovenous malformations (AVM) and dural fistulas are also usually large enough to be treated through a catheter. The choice of whether one procedure or the other, or even a combination approach, might be better for a particular patient with a particular lesion (aneurysm, AVM, dural fistula) is best made after consulting with a team of highly knowledgeable and skilled physicians that includes interventional neuroradiologists and neurosurgeons, who can properly assess the potential risks and benefits of each approach.

Leaving an Aneurysm Untreated

When an aneurysm has not ruptured, a decision must be made whether to treat it or leave it alone. Seventy percent of ruptured aneurysms result in coma or death, so treatment of an unruptured aneurysm is always given serious consideration. In general, aneurysms with a low risk of rupture are thought to be better left untreated. These include incidentally discovered aneurysms smaller than seven millimeters in diameter that form on anterior cerebral or posterior communicating arteries in a person with no symptoms and no personal or family history of subarachnoid hemorrhage. Since procedures to repair aneurysms are not risk-free, the decision to treat an unruptured aneurysm is based on the age of the patient, family history, and the size and location of the aneurysm.

Repairing Aneurysms

Aneurysms can be repaired through an open surgical procedure or a less-invasive, catheter-based, endovascular procedure. Surgery involves placing a small metal clip across the neck of the aneurysm to isolate it from blood flowing through the artery. Many aneurysms can also be treated by filling the interior of the aneurysm with tiny platinum coils or liquid material to isolate it from the circulation. A pipeline embolization device may also be used for this purpose.

Both surgery and interventional procedures can be used for aneurysms that have ruptured, as well as for those that have not. About 35 percent of ruptured aneurysms bleed again within two weeks. Consequently, a repair is scheduled within a day after a leak is discovered.

Choosing the Procedure

The choice of procedure—or decision whether a procedure is feasible—depends on the shape, size, and location of the aneurysm. Advances in endovascular technique allow wide-necked aneurysms to be treated with this approach. Fewer aneurysms are being treated with open surgical clipping. However, some aneurysms are best suited for clipping, so the choice of procedure should be discussed with a team of physicians who perform both techniques, to allow for proper risk assessment and an informed choice.

Fusiform aneurysms involve the entire circumference of the artery, which balloons out on all sides like a sausage. Fusiform aneurysms are not typically amenable to surgical treatment. New interventional techniques that include stenting have been attempted with some success. If the aneurysm is difficult to reach, or if the patient is in particularly poor health, any treatment may pose a greater risk than the aneurysm itself.

When a patient arrives in an emergency department with a ruptured aneurysm causing a subarachnoid hemorrhage, surgery is performed immediately, because the condition is life-threatening. If the aneurysm is discovered before it ruptures, a team of neurovascular specialists will decide whether clipping or an interventional procedure is more appropriate.

Surgical Clipping

Surgical clipping of an aneurysm is major surgery performed by a neurosurgeon. It requires opening the skull and moving aside brain tissue to access the part of the brain where the artery with the aneurysm is located.

The operation is performed under anesthesia. The head is immobilized by a device attached to the operating table. The head is shaved, and the section of the skull to be removed is chosen based on the location of the aneurysm. An area behind the hairline is usually selected to hide the scar. To limit swelling (edema) inside the brain, a tube may be inserted in the spinal canal to drain excess cerebrospinal fluid that bathes the subarachnoid space. A drug called mannitol (Osmitrol) or steroids may also be administered to reduce the risk of edema.

An incision is made in the skin and muscles of the head, which are folded back. Using a drill, the neurosurgeon makes a few small holes in the skull. A special jigsaw is inserted through the holes, and a section of the skull is cut out and placed aside. It will be replaced at the end of the operation.

BOX 4-7

Surgical Clipping of an Aneurysm

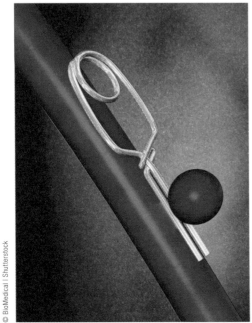

Surgical clipping requires the doctor to open up the skull and place a metal clip at the base of the aneurysm to keep it from bursting. Sometimes more than one clip is used. The procedure is done using general anesthesia, and the clip or clips are left in the body permanently.

© BioMedical I Shutterstock

BOX 4-8

Endovascular Coiling of an Aneurysm

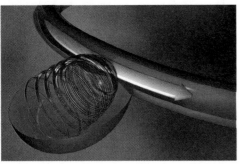

In endovascular coiling, a very thin microcatheter is inserted into the artery affected by the aneurysm. A tiny electrical current releases the coil from the catheter and into the ballooning aneurysm. The coil seals off the aneurysm from blood flow in the artery, and is left in place permanently.

© Vampy1 I Dreamstime.com

The covering of the brain (dura) is then cut and folded back. With the help of retractors, the neurosurgeon gently pushes back the brain, widening the space and creating a corridor between the brain and the skull. Using an operating microscope, the surgeon locates the artery with the aneurysm and follows it until the aneurysm is exposed.

A clip is chosen, mounted on a special instrument called a clip applier, and opened. Once it is in place around the neck of the aneurysm, the jaws are released, pinching off and isolating the aneurysm from the artery (see Box 4-7, "Surgical Clipping of an Aneurysm"). Several clips may be used. The clips remain on the artery permanently. The dome of the aneurysm is then punctured to drain it of blood.

The retractors are removed, the dura folded back over the brain and sewn closed, the skull replaced and secured with titanium plates and screws, the muscles and skin folded back into place, the incision sewn closed, and sterile surgical dressing placed over the incision. The entire operation generally takes three to five hours.

Following surgery, the patient is moved to the neurosurgical intensive care unit (NSICU) for close observation, and usually discharged after two or three days. The length of stay depends on whether the aneurysm ruptured prior to surgery.

Endovascular Treatment

Depending on the shape and location of the aneurysm and the age of the patient, an endovascular technique called coiling can be a viable treatment. Studies have shown coiling can reduce the long-term risk of death by an average of 23 percent, compared with surgery.

In coiling, a microcatheter is inserted into an artery in the groin and threaded up to the aneurysm. When the catheter tip is positioned inside the aneurysm, tiny platinum coils are deposited inside the aneurysm until the space has been filled and is no longer visible on fluoroscopy (see Box 4-8, "Endovascular Coiling of an Aneurysm"). The deposition of onyx liquid material within the aneurysm by a similar technique will achieve similar results.

Endovascular treatment is a widely accepted minimally invasive method of treating both ruptured and unruptured intracranial aneurysms. The choice between endovascular treatment and surgical clipping is made on a case-by-case basis, taking into consideration the patient's age, medical condition, and aneurysm shape and location.

Coiling combined with stenting is a minimally invasive method of treating wide-neck and some fusiform aneurysms. When an aneurysm has no neck, it is difficult to keep the coils from spilling out of the aneurysm into the artery. Placing a stent in the artery across the mouth of the aneurysm prevents this, isolating the aneurysm from the artery to prevent it from rupturing. Some fusiform aneurysms are now treated by expanding a stent across the entire length of the aneurysm and inserting coils behind the stent, which acts as a barricade to hold them in place.

Despite the initial success of coiling, up to 20 percent of patients need additional treatment. In some patients, the coils become compacted and pull away from the wall of the aneurysm, enabling blood to re-enter the defect. To monitor for this occurrence, patients are typically scheduled for an angiogram or magnetic resonance angiography (MRA) six to 12 months after coiling. If the coils have compacted, additional coils are inserted into the aneurysm.

Flow Diversion

Flow diversion is a relatively new technique that is now widely used instead of bypass surgery for treating giant aneurysms in the internal carotid arteries (see Box 4-9, "Aneurysm Flow Diversion"). Flow diverters are similar to stents. One or more may be inserted inside the blood vessel to wall off the aneurysm, essentially forming a barricade that diverts blood away from the sac. Without the pressure of blood flowing through it, the aneurysm is no longer at risk for rupture.

Other Options

There are other creative approaches to difficult-to-treat aneurysms. Two stents may be deployed in a Y configuration to treat wide-necked aneurysms that form where the two posterior cerebral arteries branch off the basilar artery (basilar apex or bifurcation aneurysms). In this procedure, called stent-assisted

BOX 4-9

Aneurysm Flow Diversion

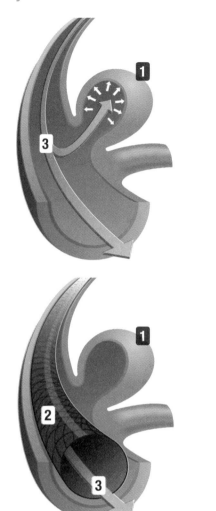

© Rob3000 | Dreamstime.com

1 Aneurysm   **2** Flow Diverter   **3** Blood flow

In aneurysm flow diversion, a stent (flow diverter) is placed in an artery with a catheter. The stent is placed so that it covers the opening to the aneurysm and keeps blood from entering the aneurysm.

coil embolization, the first stent is deployed in one of the posterior cerebral arteries at the junction. The second stent is passed through the first stent and deployed in the other posterior cerebral artery, connecting the two stents to form a Y. After both stents are in place, coils are inserted into the aneurysm to obliterate it.

Arteriovenous Malformations

Arteriovenous malformations (AVMs) are tangles of blood vessels with weak walls that are prone to rupture. While the risk of hemorrhage is only two to four percent, the fatality rate is 10 to 15 percent. The 30-year risk of having at least one bleeding episode is about 70 percent.

Doctors agree that the 10 percent of patients with symptomatic AVMs should be treated with one of three interventional treatments: surgery, closing off the vessels with glue (embolization), or destroying the blood vessels with radiation (stereotactic radiotherapy). These may be used alone or in combination.

They are not in agreement that the 90 percent of patients with asymptomatic AVMs that are discovered accidentally should be treated. The ARUBA trial demonstrated that medical management alone is superior to medical management plus interventional therapy for preventing death or stroke for up to three years in patients with unruptured brain AVMs.

If an AVM is not leaking, there is some risk that surgery might cause a leakage, so doctors must determine whether to recommend surgical or interventional treatment. The Cleveland Clinic Cerebrovascular Center has experts that specialize in all three treatment options, and often utilize a combination approach to obliterate AVMs.

EMERGENCY TREATMENT FOR STROKE

If you think you are having a stroke, call 911 immediately, or have someone close to you make the call. The ambulance will take you to the nearest hospital with a stroke center or, if there is no stroke center in your area, to the nearest Emergency Department (see Box 5-1, "The Value of a Stroke Center"). Some hospitals that are not stroke centers may still have the ability to offer specialized stroke care using specialists in another location through a video link (see Box 5-2, "What is a Telestroke Program?" on page 70). Because the speed with which you are diagnosed and treated may make the difference between a lasting disability or death and a partial or complete recovery, it is critical that you be rapidly and correctly evaluated, diagnosed, and treated. Stroke centers understand this and are prepared to take immediate action when a stroke is suspected.

The first goal is to confirm the suspected diagnosis based solely on symptoms. While this is being done, an ECG will be taken to monitor your heart rate and watch for any abnormalities or arrhythmias. Your blood pressure will be monitored and you will be given oxygen if your blood oxygen levels are lower than normal.

Diagnostic Tests and Treatment

When a stroke is suspected, imaging the brain can help differentiate whether it is ischemic or hemorrhagic in origin. This information is necessary, because the two types of stroke are treated differently. Brain imaging is usually done with computed tomography (CT). Some hospitals use magnetic resonance imaging (MRI), but the technology is too slow to use when seconds count.

CT scans enable doctors to see the brain, bones, and blood vessels with astonishing clarity. The scanner is a rotating X-ray machine that swings completely around the patient. Hundreds of X-ray images taken from all different angles are analyzed by a computer and reconstructed into images.

Bone is dense, so it absorbs X-rays well. In a brain CT scan, the skull appears white. Fluids absorb fewer X-rays, so blood vessels

BOX 5-1

The Value of a Stroke Center

Hospital stroke centers are well qualified to evaluate, diagnose, and treat stroke patients very quickly. Stroke centers always have a radiologist and neurologist on call to help the emergency physician make the proper diagnosis, determine appropriate treatment, and take immediate action. Stroke centers have a computed tomography (CT) scanner available to assist with the diagnosis, and a neurosurgeon standing by in case surgery is needed. Most stroke centers undergo a certification procedure to ensure that they are capable of and fully equipped to handle any stroke emergency. In fact, certified stroke centers are three times more likely to administer time-critical clot-busting treatment for strokes than noncertified hospitals.

Hospitals that can provide lifesaving stroke treatment, but do not have the services of a stroke center in place, are less likely to provide stroke victims with timely care. A study presented at the 2014 International Stroke Conference found that although 80 percent of people in the U.S. live within one hour of a hospital equipped to provide thrombolytic therapy for stroke, only four percent of patients receive the treatment. In fact, 63 percent of U.S. hospital did not administer a single dose of tPA in 2011, although they treated 20 percent of all stroke patients. That's why it is in your best interests to know where the closest stroke center is located, and—if you are able to—tell the paramedics to take you there.

BOX 5-2

What Is a Telestroke Program?

Many hospitals in smaller communities, especially in rural areas, lack the capability to keep highly specialized medical personnel ready to quickly assess and treat patients who arrive at the hospital with a stroke. One solution is to use telemedicine to assist with stroke care.

A telestroke program allows highly specialized experts located at stroke centers to remotely assess patients at hospitals that are not stroke centers, direct treatment and determine who qualifies for tPA. Results of imaging studies are instantly transmitted to these specialists, who consult with the on-site physicians and talk to patients via video conferencing. Because there are not enough stroke specialists to go around, and many hospitals are lucky to have a single stroke doctor on board, telestroke programs can provide coverage when their own stroke specialist is unavailable.

BOX 5-3

CT Showing Area of Damage From Hemorrhagic Stroke

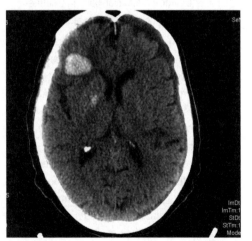

Computed tomography (CT) is usually the first type of imaging done when a hemorrhagic stroke is suspected, because it clearly shows what's happening in and around the brain. In the image above, the white areas show the damage from excessive bleeding.

and the fluid-filled subarachnoid space appear black. Brain tissue and artery walls are of an intermediate density, so they appear gray. Most areas of ischemic stroke are less dense than normal brain tissue, so they appear as dark patches in areas that should be uniformly gray. Hemorrhaged blood is dense and appears white in areas that should be darker (see Box 5-3, "CT Showing Area of Damage From Hemorrhagic Stroke").

CT scans are reliable, but they cannot show a stroke that is very small. The area affected by a stroke may not appear abnormal on CT for several hours. Additionally, CT does not image every area of the brain equally well. In an emergency, however, a CT scan can be performed and interpreted quickly.

Emergency Medical Treatment

Knowing a patient's vital signs, and armed with the results of a CT scan, ECG, blood tests, and history of stroke symptoms including time of onset, a physician can make a diagnosis. If the diagnosis is ischemic stroke, and less than 4.5 hours have elapsed since the onset of symptoms, a powerful medication called tPA may be used to dissolve the clot and restore blood flow (see Box 5-4, "Guidelines Loosened for Who Should Get tPA," on page 71). This technique is called intravenous thrombolysis—in lay terms, "clot-busting."

For patients diagnosed with ischemic stroke after the treatment window has passed, no medication to restore blood flow has been proven effective. However, some patients may benefit from mechanical clot removal (see pages 74 and 75) up to six hours after stroke onset. Further treatment is aimed at stabilizing the patient and preventing stroke progression.

It's clear that one answer is to shorten the length of time before the patient is diagnosed with stroke. Recognizing that minutes matter, medical centers like Cleveland Clinic are equipping ambulances to deliver ER services faster (see Box 5-5, "Cleveland Clinic Brings the ER to the Patient," on page 72).

Standard Treatment: Dissolve the Blood Clot

Thrombolysis is the combination of two Greek words, "thrombus," meaning blood clot, and "lysis," meaning to dissolve or break apart. The body has a natural mechanism for doing this through proteins that circulate in the blood. One of these is plasminogen, an inactive protein that the body converts to plasmin, an enzyme that breaks apart and dissolves blood clots. To make this conversion, another enzyme called tissue plasminogen activator (tPA) is required.

Blood clotting is a dynamic process. Fibrin filaments act like nets to trap red blood cells and stop the bleeding. As fibrin filaments form, tPA in the serum of the trapped blood begins to adhere to the fibrin, converting plasminogen to plasmin. Plasmin attacks the fibrin filaments, dissolving the net and breaking up the blood clot.

Blood clots are broken apart by plasmin as they form. So long as there is sufficient stimulus for blood to clot, clots will form faster than plasmin can break them apart. When the stimulus vanishes, the blood clot eventually breaks apart and disappears. The objective of thrombolytic therapy is to accelerate the removal of a blood clot by enhancing the conversion of inactive plasminogen to clot-busting plasmin.

The intravenous (IV) administration of tPA—meaning it is injected into a vein—is such an effective treatment for acute ischemic stroke that it is used in emergency departments throughout the country. Newer options include intra-arterial administration of tPA and mechanical removal of blood clots.

Several tPA drugs are used to break up heart attack-causing blood clots in the coronary arteries, but only one is approved for the treatment of ischemic stroke: alteplase (Activase). Initially, it was thought alteplase had to be administered within three hours of stroke onset. But when clinical trials showed the drug was safe and effective for a longer period of time, the American Heart Association/American Stroke Association (AHA/ASA) endorsed expanding the treatment window to 4.5 hours. However, the AHA/ASA continues to emphasize that results are better when patients are treated earlier. Patients who receive the therapy within 90 minutes have a better outcome than those who receive it later, even if within the allowed time period. For every 30 minutes that pass before blood flow is restored through a blocked artery, the probability of a good recovery drops by about 10 percent.

Alteplase is given by intravenous infusion. About 10 percent

Guidelines Loosened for Who Should Get tPA

An injection of tPA can save a life and restore quality of life. But only about five percent of patients with ischemic stroke receive the treatment. One reason is failure to arrive at the hospital within the treatment window. But other reasons involve eligibility and exclusion criteria.

The American Heart Association/American Stroke Association (AHA/ASA) took a close look at these criteria and how they fit with common practice. For example, the drug label says that risks are increased when the drug is used in patients over age 75, and its effectiveness in those over age 80 has not been established. The AHA/ASA gave a positive recommendation to tPA use in older patients, acknowledging that risk may be increased, but that risk does not outweigh the potential benefit in increasing the likelihood of remaining independent at three months after a stroke.

This is only one example of how the exclusion criteria are becoming less rigid. The AHA/ASA hope their guidelines will make physicians less reluctant to offer tPA when a patient with stroke symptoms comes to the Emergency Department.

Stroke, December 22, 2015

BOX 5-5

Cleveland Clinic Brings the ER to the Patient

Cleveland Clinic is among the first medical centers in the U.S. with mobile stroke treatment units. Both units have their own lab, CT scanner, and specially trained personnel, who diagnose and begin treatment of potential stroke patients at the scene of symptom onset and en route to the hospital in Cleveland, Ohio. Since the first unit was launched in 2014, the concept has been improved with innovations that include the use of telemedicine to allow neurologists to manage stroke cases remotely. The mobile units enable caregivers to treat patients with intravenous tPA or interventional techniques far sooner than would be possible using current standard protocols, thereby improving patient outcomes.

Cleveland Clinic Cerebrovascular Center

of the entire dose is given at one time (bolus), with the remaining 90 percent infused over an hour.

Know the Risks

A danger of thrombolytic therapy is the possibility of bleeding. Clot-busting drugs cannot tell the difference between a "bad" clot that prevents blood flow to the brain cells and a "good" clot that has been formed to stop blood flow from a ruptured intracranial artery. If the drug breaks down a good clot, a hemorrhagic stroke can occur. Despite careful dosing, intracranial hemorrhage occurs in some patients who receive alteplase. Nevertheless, in appropriately selected patients, the benefits far outweigh this potential complication.

Enhancing Clot Busting With Ultrasound

Ultrasound is often used to assess blood flow through arteries in the brain blocked by plaque or blood clots. The probe is positioned on the temporal bone of the skull, in front of and slightly above the ear. The probe acts as a transmitter and receiver of high-frequency sound waves.

Ultrasonography may have a role beyond diagnosis and may actually enhance the effect of clot-dissolving treatment. Several studies have shown that ultrasonography in addition to a clot-dissolving drug results in improved survival and greater chance for opening blocked blood vessels without increased risk for bleeding in the brain. More research is needed with this approach before it can be considered for routine use.

Endovascular Interventions

Endovascular interventions are designed to dissolve or otherwise eliminate blood clots by gaining access directly to the clot. These techniques use a catheter (a long, thin tube) that is inserted into an artery in the groin and then advanced to the location in the brain with the blood clot. This allows clot-busting drugs to be delivered directly to the blood clot, or the clot to be mechanically removed.

Delivering Medication Directly into the Brain

Delivering a clot-busting drug by catheter into an artery in the brain near or at the blood clot is called intra-arterial thrombolysis, or IAT. Early research indicated that intra-arterial delivery of clot-busting drugs may be so effective that up to 25 percent of patients experience unexpected and significant improvement—the seemingly miraculous "Lazarus phenomenon."

IAT is likely effective because delivering the drug directly to the blood clot concentrates the clot-dissolving power where it is needed most. This prevents the drug from being diluted by the blood, which occurs when a thrombolytic agent is administered into a vein in the arm. Ideally, IAT would reduce the risk of hemorrhage, since the drug's power would not be felt in the other intracranial arteries.

Several researchers have reported some success with this approach. The largest of the small clinical trials, initiated at Cleveland Clinic, tested a clot-busting drug called recombinant pro-urokinase (r-proUK). They found that patients who were treated with the medication had a 40 percent chance of regaining functional independence, compared with only 25 percent in the placebo arm, despite a higher rate of bleeding complications in the r-proUK group (10 percent vs two percent).

The use of intra-arterial thrombolysis is currently recommended only for carefully selected patients who can receive the treatment within six hours of the onset of stroke symptoms and are not candidates for intravenous tPA.

Mechanical Clot Removal

In addition to being dissolved, clots may be removed with catheter-based devices in a technique called thrombectomy. The approach has several potential advantages, including potential reduction in the risk of intracranial hemorrhage, restoration of blood flow more quickly than drugs, and, theoretically, longer effectiveness after the stroke occurs.

Four studies presented at the International Stroke Conference in 2015 showed that mechanical thrombectomy has dramatic effects. In all studies, thrombectomy significantly increased the proportion of patients who recovered well enough to live independently. One researcher said, "The trials change everything. We are now obliged to use this technology in eligible stroke patients with large-vessel occlusion. There is absolutely no question that mechanical thrombectomy should now be standard of care." Like tPA, the sooner mechanical clot removal is performed, the more impressive the results. Benefit was seen up to six hours after stroke onset.

Four different devices can be used to remove a clot:

MERCI Retriever

The MERCI Retriever is inserted in an artery, where it can be maneuvered directly to a clot that is blocking blood flow, capture it and remove it. (MERCI stands for Mechanical Embolus Removal in Cerebral Ischemia.) The device is a nitinol wire that spontaneously assumes a corkscrew shape as it moves toward the clot. The first few loops of the spiral are deployed beyond the clot, and the last loops are deployed within the clot to ensnare it (see Box 5-6, "The MERCI Retriever").

Retrievable Stents

Two clot-removing devices use retrievable stents to extract blood clots: the Solitaire Flow Restoration Device (see Box 5-7, "The Solitaire Stent Retriever," on page 75) and the Trevo Retriever. A stent is a small mesh tube that can be used to open a narrowed artery. The Solitaire and Trevo devices consist of a stent on the end of a thin catheter, which is threaded through an artery to the location of the blood clot. The clot is trapped in the stent, which is then removed. This restores blood flow through the artery.

BOX 5-6

The MERCI Retriever

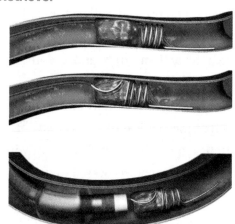

A corkscrew device is maneuvered to the blood clot, captures the clot, and removes it, restoring blood flow to the artery.

Studies comparing use of the retrievable stents with use of the Merci Retriever have favored the retrievable stents. In fact, all positive studies on thrombectomy presented at the 2015 International Stroke Conference utilized the Solitaire device.

Penumbra System

A mechanical device called the Penumbra System removes blood clots by aspiration. The technique involves delivering a catheter into the clot and using continuous suction to remove the clot.

Treating Hemorrhagic Stroke

When a hemorrhagic stroke occurs, the goal of the emergency care is to stabilize the patient and manage blood pressure by keeping it within certain limits and avoiding sudden fluctuations. If pressure inside the brain increases along with other measures, a drug called mannitol (Osmitrol) may be given to alleviate the swelling and reduce the pressure while surgical treatment is discussed.

For intracerebral or subarachnoid hemorrhage, there is no emergency treatment available to stop the bleeding. There is some potential in a surgical procedure in which a dime-sized hole is cut in the skull, a catheter is inserted into a cerebrospinal fluid-filled cavity deep in the brain, and tPA is

BOX 5-7

The Solitaire Stent Retriever

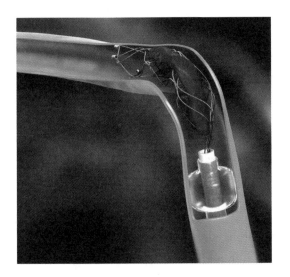

The Solitaire stent retriever is a thin, flexible device with a mesh tip that can grab a clot and pull it from an artery. It can also deliver medication to clot to help dissolve it. The retriever is used to restore blood flow through a blocked artery.

Image courtesy of Covidien Medtronic

delivered through the catheter to rapidly remove the blood from the ventricle and subarachnoid space. However, further study is required to assess if this technique improves clinical outcomes.

After an aneurysmal subarachnoid hemorrhage, there is a 30 percent chance of having another within one month. Surgical or interventional treatment of the aneurysm can lower the likelihood it will rupture again to less than one percent per year.

For patients with intracerebral hemorrhage, a clinical trial is evaluating whether aspirating the clot using a minimally invasive technique, and delivering tPA directly into the hemorrhage over three days, will improve outcomes. The trial, known as Minimally Invasive Surgery Plus rt-PA for ICH Evacuation, Phase III (MISTIE III), is expected to wrap up in 2019. It is hoped that the procedure will improve patients' long-term quality of life.

Neuroprotection

There are two aspects to stroke treatment: Treating the cause of the problem—for example, using thrombolytic therapy to restore blood flow after an ischemic stroke—and protecting the neurons from damage during the stroke. Over the years, numerous attempts to develop a neuroprotective drug have been tried and failed, although relieving pressure in the brain does offer some protection against damage from swelling. In some cases, temporary removal of a section of skull (hemicraniotomy) is performed to relieve the swelling.

Interestingly, one of the most successful neuroprotectants comes directly from Mother Nature: cold. For years, doctors have taken advantage of the fact that brain cells suffer less injury during open-heart surgery when they are cooled below normal body temperature. Difficulties inducing and managing hypothermia during the acute phase of stroke management may prevent its widespread use. However, doctors are working to develop techniques to safely induce mild hypothermia for extended periods through the use of such devices as stroke "caps" that cool the brain.

Further Testing

By the time a patient is stabilized, the doctors may know what caused the stroke. If not, additional tests may be recommended. These tests may be used to plan rehabilitation and determine eligibility for an interventional or surgical procedure to clean out any plaque in the carotid arteries, widen the arteries, or repair an aneurysm or arteriovenous malformation.

Magnetic Resonance Imaging (MRI)

Magnetic resonance imaging (MRI) is useful in all phases of stroke management, since it can identify small strokes not seen on computed tomography (CT). However, it is more expensive than CT, takes longer to perform than CT, and the equipment is not always available during an emergency.

MRI is a safe, painless, non-invasive technology that uses a large magnet turned on and off to generate movement in the atoms of the human body. As the atoms move, they emit radio signals. Different kinds of tissue emit different signals, which are captured by a computer and translated into remarkably clear images in two or three dimensions.

MRI can detect many types of brain and blood vessel abnormalities. and precisely map the area of brain tissue damaged by an ischemic stroke. Diffusion-weighted MRI is especially useful in detecting ischemic and infarcted areas of the brain soon after an ischemic stroke occurs. Gradient-echo MRI is particularly well suited for diagnosing and following the progression of cerebral amyloid angiopathy, a condition that causes tiny bleeds to occur over a period of years.

MRI can also be used to obtain detailed images of arteries in the brain and neck. This type of MRI, called magnetic resonance angiography (MRA), is used to evaluate the presence and position of plaque and blood clots in the intracranial arteries and neck arteries. It is often used prior to an interventional procedure or surgery.

Cerebral Angiography

Cerebral angiography remains the gold standard for visualizing arteries of the head and neck before a surgical procedure and before and during an interventional procedure. In this technique, X-rays are used to detect a radio-opaque contrast material injected into the arteries.

Carotid Ultrasound

Carotid ultrasound (also called carotid Doppler or carotid duplex) uses ultrasound waves produced by a hand-held transducer to assess the amount of blockage in the carotid arteries by detecting the speed of blood. The direction and flow of blood affects the reflection of sound waves, and the transducer has a receiver that detects these sounds. A computer converts the sounds into an image called a sonogram, which enables the doctor to see the arteries and hear the blood as it flows through them. A sonogram can detect plaques in carotid arteries and estimate the extent of a blockage by measuring how fast blood flows past the occlusion. Non-invasive and painless, carotid ultrasonography is virtually risk-free.

What Next?

After the crisis has passed, the patient and doctor need to discuss the chances of a complete recovery. The earlier rehabilitation begins, the better these chances are. More than likely, rehabilitation will be started immediately in the hospital.

AFTER A STROKE

Most strokes cause a neurological deficit—for example, loss of the ability to think clearly, understand, speak, or move a limb. Since memory, vision, movement, and other functions are located in specific areas of the brain, the problems experienced after a stroke depend on the area of the brain the stroke affects (see Box 6-1, "The Brain Is Neatly Compartmentalized").

The severity of a stroke depends on its size and location. The severity of an ischemic stroke also depends on how long blood flow to the brain remains blocked. When an insufficient amount of oxygenated blood is delivered to the brain for as little as 10 seconds, brain cells begin to fail. If blood flow is quickly restored, the brain cells can fully recover. After several minutes without

BOX 6-1

The Brain Is Neatly Compartmentalized

Different parts of the brain are responsible for different functions. The location of a stroke determines the symptoms the patient experiences.

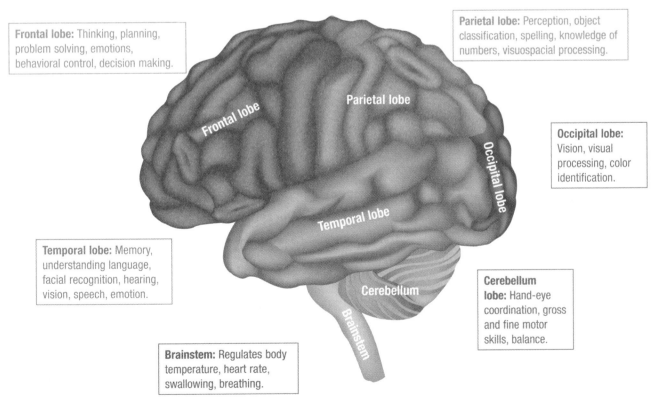

Frontal lobe: Thinking, planning, problem solving, emotions, behavioral control, decision making.

Parietal lobe: Perception, object classification, spelling, knowledge of numbers, visuospacial processing.

Occipital lobe: Vision, visual processing, color identification.

Temporal lobe: Memory, understanding language, facial recognition, hearing, vision, speech, emotion.

Cerebellum lobe: Hand-eye coordination, gross and fine motor skills, balance.

Brainstem: Regulates body temperature, heart rate, swallowing, breathing.

© Terriana | Dreamstime.com

BOX 6-2

Vagal Nerve Stimulation Shows Promise

Weakness is common after a stroke. Stimulating the vagus nerve, which connects to the brainstem, appears to cause acetylcholine and other pro-neuroplastic stimulators to be released and flood the cerebral cortex. If this is timed to occur during movements, it improves limb function. British researchers recruited 20 patients who had experienced a stroke approximately two years prior and were still having moderately severe arm dysfunction. The vagal nerve stimulator was implanted, and the patients underwent regular physical therapy sessions for six weeks. The stimulator was activated in half the patients. Function was improved enough in those who received vagal nerve stimulation during their sessions, that the researchers feel the concept should be explored in a larger trial.

adequate blood flow, however, some cells may never recover. The longer they are deprived of oxygen, the more likely they will die. Doctors call the area affected by an ischemic stroke an infarction.

Adding insult to injury, the capillaries swell when their supply of oxygenated blood is interrupted. This can prevent red blood cells from squeezing through, even after the blockage has been removed, and blood flow is restored. Doctors call this the "no-reflow phenomenon." In addition, blood vessels and capillaries lose their integrity and become more permeable when blood flow is stopped. This allows proteins, salts, and water in the blood to leak out into the brain tissue, causing brain swelling (edema). Edema evolves relatively slowly, but may complicate recovery and contribute to the overall extent of brain injury. Edema usually peaks two to four days after the initial stroke and subsides over the ensuing week or two.

With a hemorrhagic stroke, the severity depends on the amount of blood that leaks into brain tissue, how long it remains there, and where it is located. If the rupture is small, the artery will seal itself before a damaging amount of blood has leaked out. After the hemorrhage stops, the body's scavenger cells (macrophages) clean up the spilled blood. If a significant amount of blood has been released, however, delicate brain tissue can die.

Subarachnoid hemorrhagic strokes can cause cerebrospinal fluid to accumulate in the subarachnoid space (hydrocephalus). Hydrocephalus usually develops several days or weeks after a stroke, and causes increased pressure that produces a variety of symptoms: excruciating headache with nausea and vomiting; vision disorders; problems with balance, walking, and coordination; urinary incontinence; lethargy and drowsiness; and changes in personality or cognition, such as irritability and memory loss. Hydrocephalus can clear spontaneously or require the placement of a shunt, which drains the excess fluid into the abdomen.

The Road to Improvement

If you're fortunate, you'll be among the 14 percent of stroke survivors who recover fully and are able to resume their normal daily activities.

More than likely, you will be left with some residual

BOX 6-3

impairment that may make your usual activities difficult or impossible to resume. With the help of rehabilitation and medications, you will likely regain some lost function in the days and weeks after your stroke. One study found that patients who used the antidepressant drug fluoxetine (Prozac) for 90 days after a stroke had better recovery of their motor skills compared to those, taking a placebo.

In general, the rate of improvement will begin to slow down after about three months, at which time you'll have gained back much of what will return spontaneously. However, improvement may continue long after this time period (see Box 6-2, "Vagal Nerve Stimulation Shows Promise," on page 80).

One study found that hand-grip exercises started more than six months after a stroke could significantly increase activity in the area of the brain corresponding with hand use. The fact that the brain continues to adapt for longer periods of time means that retraining for loss of verbal or memory deficiencies, for example, might be possible. Another study found that walking on a treadmill any time after a stroke—even years after—significantly improved health and mobility.

Although the length of time you will need to recover depends on the severity of your stroke, you can help yourself by beginning a rehabilitation program as soon as your doctor allows you to start. Most likely, you will be given some rehabilitation in the hospital within days after your stroke. Before you are discharged, you will be given advice on where to go to continue outpatient rehabilitation. Do it! If you actively participate in a program designed for you, you can regain more of your lost function than if you do not pursue rehabilitation.

Depression is a common side effect of a stroke. Whether depression results from the injury to the brain itself or is a response to the tremendous changes patients often face after a stroke is not clear. Regardless of the cause, depression can interfere with your recovery. If you suspect you are suffering from depression, tell your doctor. Medications can be helpful, as can counseling. Some stroke survivors are at increased risk of stroke-related dementia, which can be intertwined with depression (see Box 6-3 "The Relationship of Multi-Infarct Dementia to Stroke").

The Relationship of Multi-Infarct Dementia to Stroke

Multi-infarct dementia is caused by multiple strokes or disruption of blood flow to the brain, and is a common cause of memory loss in the elderly. Here's what happens: A disruption of blood flow causes damaged brain tissue. Over time, as more areas of the brain are damaged and more small blood vessels are blocked, the symptoms of multi-infarct dementia appear.

Multi-infarct dementia typically strikes people ages 60-75 and affects more men than women. High blood pressure increases its likelihood. The symptoms of multi-infarct dementia are similar to Alzheimer's disease and as a result, it can be difficult to make a definitive diagnosis. Retinal circulation in the eye allows doctors to non-invasively detect evidence of cerebral microvascular disease. People with signs of retinopathy, such as microaneurysms or retinal hemorrhages, may be more likely to also have cognitive impairment.

Multi-Infarct Dementia is Marked by:
- Confusion
- Walking with rapid, shuffling steps
- Problems with short-term memory
- Laughing or crying inappropriately
- Wandering
- Difficulty following instructions
- Getting lost in familiar places
- Urinary incontinence
- Problems counting money and making monetary transactions.

Multi-infarct dementia can be confirmed with magnetic resonance imaging (MRI) or computed tomography (CT) imaging, along with a neurological examination.

Unfortunately, there are no treatments to reverse brain damage that has been caused by a stroke. Instead, treatment focuses on preventing future strokes by controlling risk factors, including high blood pressure, diabetes, high cholesterol, and heart disease.

Although you cannot change the extent of your brain injury, there are things you can do to help yourself recover. First, start rehabilitation early. Second, adopt a positive attitude and believe in yourself. Third, follow the advice and recommendations of your rehabilitation team. Fourth, ask your family and friends to give you encouragement, help, and support. You may not be able to regain all of your abilities, but even an incremental improvement can make the difference between being able to return home or needing assisted living.

Most importantly, do everything you can to prevent a second stroke by taking recommended medications faithfully, and making suggested lifestyle changes to decrease your risk. These steps will be explained later in this chapter.

Researchers are studying stem cell therapy and other new approaches that might help the brain repair itself after a stroke. These investigations are in their very early stages, but they hold promise for faster, more complete recovery from stroke

Committing to Rehabilitation

Rehabilitation is a long-term process designed to help you improve your physical and mental capabilities and adjust to your disabilities. It is essential in helping you maintain your strength and confidence. The goal of rehabilitation is to make you as independent and productive as you can be, and help you achieve the best possible quality of life.

If certain functions have been lost, new ones can be learned through repetition. This helps the brain reestablish lost connections by rerouting nerve signals or training another part of your body to assume the lost function. Different rehabilitation programs focus on different goals, and rehabilitation experts use very modern techniques to help patients restore lost function. For example, in some cases video games and smartphone and tablet applications are used to help improve the fine motor function needed to perform activities of daily living. Studies have shown how focused efforts can improve outcomes.

Rehabilitation Goals

The rehabilitation process begins by assessing your disabilities and lost skills (see Box 6-4, "Lost Functions and Skills," on page 83). The information will be used to design a rehabilitation plan to address your specific needs. The plan will be based on your ability to:

- Take care of yourself by eating, grooming, bathing, dressing, and going to the toilet.
- Get around by yourself, either by walking or in a self-propelled wheelchair, and change positions, for example, rising from a chair or bed.
- Communicate by speaking, reading, writing, or using a computer.
- Remember new events and learn new facts or to recall memories.
- Solve problems.
- Interact appropriately with other people in private and in public.

BOX 6-4

Lost Functions and Skills

Stroke survivors who do not fully recover will experience one or more of the disabilities cited below. Most of these disabilities are extensions of the stroke survivor's first symptoms. Lasting disabilities can be grouped in five categories:

❶ Movement

- Weakness (hemiparesis) or paralysis (hemiplegia) on one side of the body.
- Uncontrollable muscle tightness and stiffness (post-stroke spasticity), which causes painful muscle cramps in the arms and legs.
- Inability to maintain balance.
- Inability to coordinate movements (ataxia).
- Trouble swallowing food or drinks (dysphagia).

❷ Sensation

- Inability to feel touch, pain, heat, cold or position.
- Feeling pain, numbness or odd sensations like pins and needles on the weak or paralyzed side (paresthesia).
- Inability to control the bowels or bladder, due to loss of the sensation of the need to urinate or have a bowel movement. May also involve the inability to control the bladder or rectal muscles.
- Development of chronic pain. Neuropathic pain is due to brain damage and the generation and transmission of nerve signals that are mistakenly perceived as pain. Chronic pain may also be due to immobilization in a paralyzed joint (frozen joint).

❸ Language

- Inability or difficulty in using or understanding speech and writing (aphasia).
- Inability to speak clearly and coherently, even when the right words are known (dysarthria).

❹ Cognition

- Loss of cognitive ability, including memory, thinking, keeping attention focused (awareness), comprehension or learning.
- Inability to plan and perform a task requiring several complex steps or following instructions to perform a task (apraxia).
- Inability to understand and acknowledge any physical disabilities resulting from the stroke (anosognosia).
- Inability to respond to objects or sensations on your weak or paralyzed side (neglect).

❺ Emotion

- Feeling fear, anxiety, frustration, anger, sadness and grief. Part of this may be due to brain damage, and part due to natural response to the trauma of a stroke.
- Losing control of your emotions (emotional lability).
- Fatigue.
- Depression.

In-Hospital Rehabilitation

As soon as you have been stabilized, rehabilitation nurses will encourage you to move around, even if you are weak or partially paralyzed. They will help you change positions in bed to prevent bedsores, transfer you from the bed to a chair, and help you walk. You'll start with these simple movements and progress to more complex tasks, such as using the toilet, bathing, and dressing. Regaining your ability to do these movements may not happen right away, but you should see improvement in the first few days. As you progress and become more capable, your nurse will offer less assistance and more encouragement.

Exercising a weakened or paralyzed arm or leg is important to prevent the tendons and muscles around your joints from "freezing." Your rehabilitation nurse will move your arm or leg through its usual range of motion. These are called passive exercises. Once you are able, you'll be guided through active exercises, where you control the movements of your stroke-impaired arm or leg without assistance. These exercises will help you strengthen your limb and stay in shape, which is important for your general health and to reduce the risk of another ischemic stroke.

Rehabilitation nurses will also teach you how and when to take your medicine and care for other diseases or conditions you might have, such as diabetes or incontinence. Fortunately, stroke-related incontinence usually resolves quickly, particularly with the use of special exercises.

Prior to your discharge from the hospital, rehabilitation nurses will also play a key role in educating and training any family members, friends or companions who will be caring for you at home.

The neurologist who takes care of you while you are still in the hospital will decide when to discharge you and will give permission for your rehabilitation to start.

Rehabilitation After Hospital Discharge

Where you will undergo rehabilitation after being discharged from the hospital depends on the extent of your disability and the type of services ordered by your doctor. Post-discharge rehabilitation may be done at an outpatient rehabilitation unit connected with a hospital, or in an independent rehabilitation facility. Such facilities are staffed with the full range of rehabilitation specialists and at least one physiatrist (rehabilitation physician). Your rehabilitation will be scheduled for several hours a day at least three days a week.

Home-based rehabilitation is often arranged for stroke survivors who have no transportation to an outpatient rehabilitation unit or clinic. Although the rehabilitation specialists may not be able to provide you with the same extent of equipment found in a rehabilitation center, you'll be in a comfortable, familiar environment, and will be able to adapt what you learn to living in your home.

Rehabilitation Involves Many Specialists

The range of disabilities resulting from stroke requires different rehabilitation methods, strategies, and specialists. Many stroke survivors have multiple rehabilitation needs and see more than one rehabilitation specialist; for example, a physical therapist, occupational therapist, and speech therapist. Each type is trained in the rehabilitation of a particular type of disability using specific techniques and will help you regain as much independence as possible.

Your rehabilitation team will include some or all of the following professionals:

Physiatrists

These doctors specialize in physical medicine and rehabilitation. They focus on restoring function. Nearly every rehabilitation center has one or more physiatrists on staff.

Physical Therapists

Physical therapists are trained in the anatomy and physiology of movement and will help you improve your movement, balance and coordination. They understand the importance of building strength and endurance, as well as maintaining and extending range of motion. If you have difficulty walking, they will provide exercises to improve it. They will attempt to get the most out of your weakened or partially paralyzed limbs and teach you how to compensate for any permanent impairment. They will give you an exercise program to keep you in shape and help you retain any new skills you learn.

Physical therapists often use special facilities or equipment, such as a swimming pool. Pool exercises (hydrotherapy) are often useful in stroke survivors who can't stand on their own or can't bear their own weight. The water provides support as well as resistance to movement, and allows a much wider range of motion than lying in bed or sitting in a chair. In facilities without a swimming pool, a suspension harness may be used instead.

Your physical therapist will direct exercises designed to help you regain your ability to live independently, such as walking and climbing stairs. Most of the exercises are goal-oriented and involve hard work, but you may also have fun and stay in shape by playing games that require repetitive motion and coordination.

Occupational Therapists

Occupational therapists concentrate on the ability to perform specific tasks necessary to live independently. They may design your rehabilitation to help you function at work, do your favorite activities, cook, or drive a car. They also will teach you how to use devices that help you get around, such as a cane, walker, or wheelchair. They know many tricks of the trade—for example, substituting Velcro closures for buttons on your clothes if one of your arms is paralyzed.

Occupational therapists often break down tasks into separate steps. Practicing each step by itself before putting them together will help you master the entire task.

Occupational therapists are also trained to evaluate your home for any changes that need to be made to improve access or safety. For example, they may recommend installing ramps, removing doors, and adding grab-rails in the bathroom and shower.

Speech-Language Pathologists

Speech-language pathologists are trained to treat aphasia (the inability to communicate), one of the most frustrating consequences of many strokes. Rehabilitation may involve relearning language or using alternative means of communication such as symbol boards, sign language, or a computer. Listening to music may also help patients recover language function more quickly. Exercises in reading and writing can be important in relearning these skills, while repeating words helps in regaining the ability to speak.

Speech-language pathologists are also trained to help patients who have difficulty swallowing after a stroke (dysphagia), because swallowing and speech involve many of the same muscles. Sometimes dysphagia involves the swallowing reflex, but it may be caused by the inability to sense where food is located in the mouth. Speech-language pathologists can recommend ways to overcome these problems, and solutions may be as simple as changing posture while eating, or taking smaller bites and chewing more slowly and deliberately.

Vocational Therapists

About 25 percent of all strokes occur in people between ages 45 and 65, many of whom hope to return to their old job or, if that's not possible, learn a new skill. If your stroke occurred before retirement, then you'll probably meet with a vocational therapist. In addition to evaluating your skills and abilities, vocational therapists can serve as career counselors. They are trained to look beyond your disabilities and focus on what you can do with your strengths. They identify jobs and careers that use those skills and strengths and help you identify potential employers and write letters in support of your job application.

Vocational therapists are familiar with the legal rights of disabled people. The Americans with Disabilities Act of 1990 requires employers to make "reasonable accommodations" for disabled employees. Vocational therapists will inform you about the law so you can spot any potential violations at your workplace and discuss them with your employer. If necessary, they may act as impartial mediators to help resolve any problems.

Recreational Therapists

Recreation is important for your well-being and sense of self-esteem. Being able to enjoy recreational pursuits will go a long way in helping you get back into a normal routine, have fun and interact with other people. Many recreational activities also help you stay in shape. Recreational therapists provide advice on how to use your spare time to enhance your quality of life. They often arrange for stroke survivors to get together at events where everyone participates in activities that help maintain and improve coordination, as well as strengthen social skills and emotional stability. Recreational therapists also encourage healthy family members and friends to participate.

Music Therapists

A growing number of medical centers offer music therapy. Patients who listen to music in the weeks following a stroke show rapid increase in verbal ability and the ability to resolve conflicts and perform mental operations. In addition, they tend to be less depressed and confused.

Psychologists

Psychologists are concerned about mental and emotional health. They can help you learn how to cope with your disability and build your self-esteem. They are open to discussing family problems and other issues resulting from your stroke. Up to one-third of patients suffer depression following a stroke, and this is associated with increased disability, reduced quality of life, and increased risk of death. If the psychologist notices any signs of depression, you will be referred to a psychiatrist to discuss medication.

Nutritionists

Nutritionists may be consulted to help you modify your diet in order to reduce the risk of another stroke. They will teach you which foods to avoid and which ones to add to your diet, as well as advise you how many calories you need every day to maintain your metabolism without gaining weight.

Social Workers

You and your family may meet with a social worker while you are still in the hospital. A social worker will counsel you on your finances and advise you how to obtain help if you need it. The social worker will facilitate your transfer home and help arrange visits by rehabilitation specialists and other services, such as Meals on Wheels. He or she can help you wade through the paperwork you and your family may encounter in paying your bills, settling with your insurance company, and obtaining government assistance.

Support Groups

After a stroke, you are not alone. Many thousands of people have had the same experience. Joining a support group is something you can do to help yourself and those who help care for you.

There is a good chance one or more support groups meet regularly in your local area. Think about joining one of them (see Box 6-5, "Support Groups").

Preventing Another Stroke

About 15 percent of people who survive a stroke or TIA have a second stroke within one year—half within the first week. That's why it's critically important to take recommended medications and make lifestyle changes designed to prevent a second stroke. You are at increased risk if you have other forms of cardiovascular disease, such as coronary artery disease (CAD) or peripheral arterial disease (PAD). Stroke also increases the risk of certain medical problems, such a hip and femur fracture, so a close relationship with your primary physician is necessary to keep you healthy and out of the hospital.

If you are considering elective surgery, such as a hip or knee replacement, you would be wise to wait at least nine months—longer, if possible. A 2014 study found that patients who undergo noncardiac surgery after a stroke are at increased risk for major complications and even death, when the surgery is performed within nine months following the stroke. The researchers examined the association between stroke and noncardiac surgery in 480,000 patients, and found the risk of death within 30 days nearly doubled, and the risk of a major complication increased five-fold after a stroke. Whether the surgery was high-risk or low-risk didn't matter. The risk was highest within three months after the stroke, and leveled off after nine months, but continued to remain higher than normal.

Preventing another stroke depends heavily on taking control of the risk factors discussed in Chapter 3. Treating hypertension and LDL cholesterol is very important. Lowering systolic blood pressure (the top number) to less than 130 mmHg may reduce the risk of a second stroke by almost 20 percent. Your doctor may prescribe medication for these conditions, and you may need to change your diet. The most recent Stroke Prevention Guidelines (see Box 6-6, "Guidelines for Secondary Stroke Prevention") recommend adopting a Mediterranean diet, which emphasizes vegetables, fruits, whole grains, low-fat dairy, poultry, fish, legumes, olive oil, and nuts.

BOX 6-5

Support Groups

The American Heart Association lists stroke support groups on its website, www.americanheart.org. In the search box, type "stroke support."

You also can use the Internet to find local stroke support groups.

BOX 6-6

Guidelines for Secondary Stroke Prevention

In 2013, the American Heart Association/American Stroke Association updated their recommendations for secondary stroke prevention for survivors of ischemic stroke and TIA:

- For patients with atherosclerotic stroke or TIA and without coronary artery disease, and LDL greater than or equal to 100 mg/dl, target LDL cholesterol should be a 50 percent reduction, or less than 70 mg/dl.

- For patients with stroke or TIA and metabolic syndrome, counseling on lifestyle modification (diet, exercise, weight loss) and treatment of stroke risk factors are recommended.

- For patients with stroke or TIA and carotid artery stenosis, best medical therapy includes antiplatelet therapy, statin, and risk factor modification.

- For patients with stroke or TIA caused by a 50-99 percent blockage of a major intracranial artery, aspirin at 50-325 mg/day, rather than warfarin; blood pressure less than 140/90 mm Hg; total cholesterol less than 200 mg/dL; no extracranial or intracranial bypass surgery.

- For patients with atrial fibrillation at high risk for stroke who must temporarily stop oral anticoagulation (e.g. for surgery), use of low-molecular-weight heparin.

- For patients with atrial fibrillation who cannot take warfarin, aspirin or apixaban.

Diabetes Drug May Prevent a Second Stroke

About half of patients who suffer a stroke or TIA have insulin resistance (see page 51), but have not developed diabetes. A landmark study presented at the 2016 International Stroke Conference found the diabetes drug pioglitazone (Actos) helped these patients prevent a second stroke or heart attack. The medication also reduced the risk of developing diabetes, but did contribute to the rate of weight gain, edema, and bone fracture. This is the first time a diabetes drug has been shown to prevent heart attack and stroke.

New England Journal of Medicine, February 17, 2016

Exercise can help you lose weight, which will help resolve your metabolic syndrome or diabetes, and may be beneficial even if you don't have diabetes. If you have the heartbeat abnormality atrial fibrillation you will need to take an anticoagulant. In general, the advice for preventing a second stroke is the same as that for preventing a first stroke, and can be found in Chapter 3 and in Box 6-6, "Guidelines for Secondary Stroke Prevention," on page 89.

Your doctor will devise a medical management plan to reduce your risk of stroke. It will be up to you to follow your doctor's recommendations. One study showed that an alarmingly high number of patients fail to follow advice that could prevent another stroke. For example, 23 percent of patients in the study failed to take daily aspirin, 69 percent were not undergoing post-stroke outpatient rehabilitation, 43 percent were not getting regular exercise, 34 percent were still smoking, 19 percent were not managing their cholesterol, and nine percent were not taking medication for hypertension.

After a stroke, your doctor might prescribe aspirin or aspirin-like medications, which have been shown to reduce the risk of subsequent stroke by 20 to 25 percent. Many such agents are available, and doctors are trying to determine which ones are best for which patients.

Aspirin is one of the principal medications used to prevent a second stroke. The Food and Drug Administration recommends a daily dose of 50 to 325 mg, although the optimal dose is unknown. Because some people do not respond to aspirin, clopidogrel (Plavix) or aspirin plus extended-release dipyridamole (Permole, Persantine) may be prescribed. Your doctor is also likely to prescribe a cholesterol-lowering statin, particularly if you have diabetes or metabolic syndrome. One study showed that taking the statin drug atorvastatin (Lipitor) can prevent stroke, even in patients with metabolic syndrome or diabetes. If you have metabolic syndrome, you may benefit from a diabetes drug, even if you have not yet developed diabetes (see Box 6-7, "Diabetes Drug May Prevent a Second Stroke"). If you have symptomatic carotid artery stenosis, guidelines recommend antiplatelet therapy, a statin, and risk factor modification for prevention of another stroke.

A LAST WORD…

A stroke is a life-changing event. Yet more people than ever are surviving their stroke and going on to live happy, productive lives. Researchers have made amazing advances in preserving brain function during a stroke. They have also identified many risk factors for stroke, and have found different ways of looking inside the head and neck for structural anomalies or evidence of atherosclerosis that increases the risk for stroke. These advances, along with straightforward interventions, such as low-dose aspirin therapy, have made a difference.

Physicians and hospitals nationwide are working hard to ensure patients receive the approved treatments for stroke, no matter how big or small the hospital or where it is located. The practice of evidence-based medicine has been largely responsible for saving the lives and preserving the quality of life for countless stroke patients.

More so today than ever, people who are at risk of stroke can be identified and offered treatment before a stroke occurs (see Box 7-1, "Study Evaluates the Best Way to Prevent Stroke"). Most importantly, many Americans are taking measures to prevent a stroke, such as eating a healthier diet and exercising more. Rehabilitation techniques have also improved.

Research Continues

Important research aimed at improving care for stroke patients and survivors is underway worldwide. The problem is being approached on many fronts, including:

- Finding methods to detect the earliest signs of cerebrovascular disease.
- Using brain pattern recognition software to identify patients at increased risk of undesirable bleeding, if given tPA.
- Finding thrombolytic agents that dissolve clots faster and more effectively than tPA.
- Identifying the factors that trigger strokes.
- Understanding how the blood-brain barrier fails to prevent blood from entering the brain after a stroke.

NEW FINDING BOX 7-1

Study Evaluates the Best Way to Prevent Stroke

Even with better treatments for stroke, preventing a brain attack is still preferable. In people who have symptoms of stroke, emergency treatments such as those found in Chapter 5 can do the job. But what about people without symptoms, who are at risk?

The Carotid Revascularization and Medical Management for Asymptomatic Carotid Stenosis Study (CREST-2) is comparing three methods of stroke prevention to see which is safest and most effective. These include medical management alone, medical management plus carotid endarterectomy, and medical management plus carotid stenting. All patients in the study receive aspirin, blood pressure and cholesterol medications, and must commit to losing weight, increasing physical activity, quitting smoking and limiting alcohol use.

All study participants must have a narrowing of at least 70 percent in one or both carotid arteries, but no symptoms of TIA or stroke. They will be followed for four years. The researchers hope to have results by December 2020.

New England Journal of Medicine, March 17, 2016

- Finding a blood test that can diagnose type of stroke and assist in determining proper treatment.
- Determining the best ways to prevent lasting disabilities.
- Easing the body's response to stroke.
- Evaluating the efficacy of cooling patients' core temperature after tPA to minimize clinical deficits.
- Learning more about basic cellular changes that lead to the death of neurons after a stroke.
- Improving rehabilitation methods to help patients regain more function.
- Improving the medical, interventional, and surgical treatments for stroke.
- Assessing the value of stem cells in restoring function after stroke.

A stroke can happen to anyone at any time, but as you've just learned, there is much you can do to cut your risk of a brain attack. And if you do endure a stroke, the treatment options available to doctors are improving all the time. Indeed, the rate of fatal strokes is dropping, partly because people are living healthier lives and they're learning how to respond to stroke symptoms. But lives are also being saved because medical science advancing so rapidly. By reading this report, you've armed yourself with some invaluable knowledge. You know what to do and what to avoid to keep your brain healthy, and you can relax a little knowing how much research is ongoing to help prevent and treat strokes in the future.

**Some of the terms used in this report are frequently mentioned to stroke patients.
Always ask your doctor if you do not understand what is being said.**

Ablation: The destruction of heart tissue, usually with heat, cold, or sound waves. In patients with abnormal heart rhythms, ablation is sometimes used to destroy tissue that is causing the rhythm disturbance.

Acetylcholine: A neurotransmitter in the parts of the brain involved in thinking, learning, and memory. Neurotransmitters are chemicals that allow cells in the brain to communicate with one another.

Amyloid plaque: Protein pieces called beta-amyloid that clump together in the brains of people with Alzheimer's disease, which impairs the ability of brain cells to function properly.

Amyloid precursor protein (APP): The beta-amyloid that clumps together to form amyloid plaques is a small piece of this larger protein.

Aneurysm: An abnormal bulge in a blood vessel caused by disease or weakness of the blood vessel wall.

Angiogram: A moving X-ray image of blood flowing through coronary arteries.

Anticoagulants: Drugs that prevent blood from clotting; these include heparin and warfarin (Coumadin).

Antiplatelet agents: Drugs that inhibit the activation of platelets and, in so doing, help prevent blood from clotting; they include aspirin and clopidogrel (Plavix).

Aorta: The large, main artery exiting the heart. All blood pumped out of the left ventricle travels through the aorta on its way to other parts of the body.

Aphasia: Difficulty speaking or understanding language; difficulty reading and writing. It is caused by damage to certain areas of the brain, and can occur in people who have had a stroke, or who are in the later stages of Alzheimer's disease.

Arrhythmia: An irregular heart rate in which the heart beats too slowly, too quickly, or out of its normal rhythm.

Arteriovenous malformation: Abnormality in the structure of blood vessels; usually, a tangle of blood vessels.

Artery: Blood vessels that carry oxygenated blood from the heart to the organs and tissues.

Atherosclerosis: Narrowing of the arteries due to an accumulation of fatty deposits and plaque.

Atrial fibrillation (AF): A heart-rhythm disorder (arrhythmia) in which the upper chambers of the heart (atria) contract rapidly, creating a fast, irregular heart rhythm that weakens the heart's ability to pump.

Atrium: One of two thin-walled upper chambers of the heart that receive blood from veins. The left atrium receives oxygenated blood from the lungs; the right atrium receives oxygen-depleted blood from the body. The atria pump blood into the heart's ventricles.

Basal ganglia: Structure in the inner brain that mediates between the cerebral hemispheres and the spinal cord, and is crucial to movement.

Blood clot (see *thrombus*): A blood clot forms when clotting factors cause it to coagulate and become a jelly-like mass. When a blood clot forms inside a blood vessel (a thrombus), it can dislodge, travel through the bloodstream and become trapped, causing a heart attack or stroke.

Brainstem: The bundle of nerves at the base of the brain that allows the brain and body to communicate. The brainstem regulates basic functions such as sleep, arousal, breathing, and heart rate.

Capillaries: The smallest of the body's blood vessels that deliver nutrients and oxygen to the body's cells and remove wastes like carbon dioxide from the cells.

Cardiomyopathies: Diseases that affect the heart muscle, decreasing the ability of the heart to do its pumping job. Cardiomyopathies can be ischemic (due to coronary blockages and subsequent heart attacks) or nonischemic (from a variety of causes, including valve disease, hypertension, infiltration with iron or protein, and viruses).

Carotid artery disease: Narrowing of the major blood vessel in the neck that supplies the brain with oxygen-rich blood. It is caused by plaque buildup inside the artery walls.

Carotid endarterectomy: A surgical procedure to remove obstructive plaque in a carotid artery.

Catheter: A long, thin tube that is inserted into the arteries or veins for diagnostic or therapeutic purposes. Cardiologists can measure pressures, inject contrast dye and drugs, insert tools for measurements, and insert stents through catheters.

Cerebellum: The part of the brain related to movement, balance, and emotion.

Cerebrospinal fluid: This clear fluid acts as a cushion and surrounds the brain and spinal cord.

Cerebrum: The largest part of the brain, responsible for conscious mental processes, such as thinking, learning, and memory. The cerebrum is divided into left and right hemispheres ("left brain," "right brain").

Cholesterol: A waxy, fat-like substance found in foods of animal origin and synthesized by the body. Cholesterol is used for many of the body's processes, including hormone production. In large amounts in the blood, cholesterol can clog arteries.

Circulatory system: Composed of the heart, blood, and blood vessels (veins and arteries), the circulatory system distributes blood throughout the body. Blood that contains oxygen (oxygenated) is pumped from the lungs into the heart and out through the arteries to all parts of the body. Veins carry blood that has been depleted of oxygen back to the heart where it is pumped into the lungs to receive oxygen.

Clinical trials: Research studies that test medical treatments in humans. The optimal clinical trials are randomized, placebo-controlled studies, meaning the participants are randomly assigned to treatment groups, and one group receives a placebo (inactive pill or device) and the other receives the study drug or device. In double-blind trials, neither the researchers nor the patients know which therapy any patient has received until the study is over. This removes any chance of bias in the results.

Cognitive decline: A loss of cognitive function, such as that associated with dementia.

CT scan (computed tomography): Computer-assisted scans that can assemble a static cross-section of the brain or other internal body area using X-rays. When assembled, the images provide a three-dimensional view of the area. People suspected of having dementia may have a CT scan of the brain to look for possible alternative causes of symptoms, such as a tumor or stroke.

Diabetes: A condition in which the body does not produce or properly use the hormone insulin, which is needed to convert sugar, starches, and other food into energy. Type 1 diabetes occurs when the pancreas stops producing insulin. Type 2 diabetes occurs when cells in the body cease to respond to insulin circulating in the bloodstream.

Diastolic pressure (see *systolic pressure*): The blood pressure in the arteries when the heart is filling with blood. It is the lower of two blood pressure measurements. For example, in a blood pressure reading of 120/80 mm Hg, 80 is the diastolic pressure.

Dyspnea: Shortness of breath.

Embolic stroke: A stroke caused by a blood clot that formed elsewhere in the body, was carried into the brain by blood flow, and became stuck in an artery, effectively stopping blood flow.

Embolism: A blood clot or piece of plaque that forms elsewhere in the body and breaks away to form a blockage, unlike a thrombus, which forms a blockage at the site of origin.

Endothelial cell: The type of cell that forms the inner lining of all arteries and veins.

Endothelium: The thin layer of cells that lines the inside of blood vessels and provides a smooth surface over which blood can flow.

HDL cholesterol (see *high-density lipoprotein*): The "good" cholesterol.

Hematoma: A pool of clotted blood that has spilled out of a break in an artery or vein into tissue. In the skin, a hematoma appears as a bruise.

Hemorrhagic stroke: A stroke caused by the leakage of blood out of a blood vessel into the brain.

High blood pressure (hypertension): Blood pressure measures the force of blood against the artery walls. High blood pressure is force at an abnormally high level.

High-density lipoprotein (HDL) cholesterol: A type of "good" lipoprotein particle that carries "bad" (LDL) cholesterol to the liver, where it is processed for removal from the body. HDL-C reduces cholesterol buildup in the arteries, lowering the risk of heart attack and stroke.

Hypertension: See *high blood pressure*.

Intracerebral hemorrhage: Blood leaking from an artery into brain tissue.

Ischemia: Pronounced "iss-KEE-mee-uh," this term derives from the Greek word meaning "restriction of blood." Ischemia is a deficiency in blood flow to a tissue or organ resulting in insufficient oxygen delivery to the cells. In general, ischemia occurs during periods of increased oxygen demand (such as during exercise), and resolves with rest. The painful symptom of angina occurs due to ischemia of the heart muscle tissue.

Ischemic stroke: A stroke caused when a blocked blood vessel to the brain starves the brain tissue of oxygen.

LDL (see *low-density lipoprotein*) cholesterol: The "bad" cholesterol.

Lipid: A word used to encompass many different kinds of fat-soluble molecules, including cholesterol, triglycerides, and free fatty acids.

Lipoprotein: A specialized, microscopic, spherical particle in the blood composed of protein and lipids. Its role is to move lipids from one part of the body to another.

Low-density lipoprotein (LDL) cholesterol: A type of particle that carries cholesterol and bad fats throughout the body. LDL can build up in arteries and lead to heart attack and stroke.

Lumen: The area inside an artery or vein through which the blood flows, similar to the inside of a pipe. The lumen of the coronary artery is the only region highlighted by contrast dye during coronary angiography.

Mediterranean diet: A dietary pattern similar to that traditionally found in areas around the Mediterranean Sea in countries such as Greece, southern Italy, and Spain. It emphasizes olive oil as the primary source of dietary fat, an abundance of plant foods, including fruits, vegetables, whole grains, beans, nuts, and seeds, and moderate amounts of fish, poultry, dairy foods, and wine. The Mediterranean diet is low in red meat and saturated fats and contains no added sugars or processed foods.

Neurons: Nerve cells that transmit electrical and chemical messages via the nervous system throughout the brain, spinal cord, and body.

Palsy: Another word for a paralysis that is sometimes accompanied by involuntary tremors.

Patent: Pronounced "PAY-tunt." In medical language, this adjective means that an artery or a bypass graft is open. The noun form is "patency," pronounced "PAY-tunt-see."

Placebo: An inactive substance used in randomized, controlled scientific studies, usually when testing medications. Study participants who receive placebos are the "control group," and their data are compared with data from participants who are taking the medication being studied. However, study participants are "blind," meaning they are not told if they are taking a placebo or a medication.

Plaque (see amyloid plaque): Fatty deposits that form on the inside surface of arteries that are characteristic of atherosclerosis; plaque may contain lipids (including cholesterol), calcium, white blood cells, and blood clots.

Platelets: Small cells that circulate in the blood and help form blood clots. Medications such as aspirin, warfarin (Coumadin), and clopidogrel (Plavix) inhibit or inactivate platelets, resulting in a lower chance of blood clot formation (and a higher chance of bleeding).

Restenosis: Recurrent development of atherosclerosis at the same location, or narrowing of the blood vessel recurring at the same location where stenting or balloon angioplasty has been performed.

Revascularization: A procedure designed to restore blood flow through or around a blocked artery.

Statin: A type of drug that lowers the levels of total cholesterol and low-density lipoprotein cholesterol (LDL-C) in the blood.

Stenosis: A narrowing or constriction of a blood vessel or other opening.

Stent: A small, flexible tube made of metal mesh that can be inserted into arteries to expand narrow openings. A stent is placed in the artery by inflating a balloon (similar to those used in balloon angioplasty) that presses the wire mesh outward into the blood vessel wall.

Stroke: An acute vascular event that occurs in the brain, most often caused by a blood clot that lodges in an artery and blocks the flow of blood to the brain (ischemic stroke), producing symptoms ranging from limb paralysis and loss of speech to unconsciousness and death. Less commonly, a stroke may be caused by bleeding into the brain (hemorrhagic stroke).

Subarachnoid space: A fluid-filled space between the bones of the skull and the brain.

Systolic pressure: The pressure of the blood in the arteries when the heart contracts. It is the higher of two blood pressure measurements. For example, in a blood pressure reading of 120/80 mm Hg, 120 is the systolic pressure.

Thalamus: The part of the brain responsible for senses such as pain, burning, freezing, and itching.

Thrombolysis: The act of breaking apart or dissolving a blood clot.

Thrombosis (see *blood clot*): A blood clot inside a blood vessel.

Thrombotic stroke: A stroke resulting when a blood clot (thrombus) stops the flow of blood in an artery leading to or in the brain.

Transient ischemic attack (TIA): Occurs when blood flow to a certain part of the brain is cut off for a short period of time. It's a warning sign that something is wrong, and that a full-blown stroke could be imminent.

Vasospasm: A blood vessel spasm that causes the blood vessel to narrow and restrict blood flow.

Veins: These are blood vessels that carry deoxygenated blood back toward the heart and lungs.

Ventricles: The thick, muscular, lower chambers of the heart that pump blood out of the heart into arteries. The right ventricle pumps blood through the pulmonary artery to the lungs; the left ventricle pumps blood to the aorta for delivery to the rest of the body.

Useful organizations for information and support:

American Academy of Physical Medicine and Rehabilitation
www.aapmr.org
877-227-6799
info@aapmr.org
9700 W. Bryn Mawr Avenue, Suite 200
Rosemont, IL 60618

Academy of Nutrition and Dietetics
www.eatright.org
800-877-1600
120 South Riverside Plaza, Suite 2000
Chicago, IL 60606-6995

American Occupational Therapy Association
www.aota.org
301-652-6611
4720 Montgomery Lane, Suite 200
Bethesda, MD 20814-3449

American Physical Therapy Association
www.apta.org
800-999-2782
1111 N. Fairfax Street
Alexandria, VA 22314-1488

American Speech-Language-Hearing Association (ASHA)
www.asha.org
800-638-8255
2200 Research Boulevard
Rockville, MD 20850-3289

American Stroke Association
www.strokeassociation.org
888-4-STROKE (888-478-7653)
7272 Greenville Avenue
Dallas, TX 75231

Easter Seals
www.easterseals.com
800-221-6827
233 S. Wacker Drive; Suite 2400
Chicago, IL 60606

National Aphasia Association
www.aphasia.org
800-922-4622
naa@aphasia.org

National Heart, Lung and Blood Institute (NHLBI)
www.nhlbi.nih.gov/
301-592-8573
NHLBI Health Information Center
P.O. Box 30105
Bethesda, MD 20824-0105
  Cholesterol education:
  www.nhlbi.nih.gov/health/resources/heart#chol

National Institute on Disability, Independent Living, and Rehabilitation Research (NIDILRR)
www.acl.gov/programs/NIDILRR/
202-245-7640
nidrr-mailbox@ed.gov

National Rehabilitation Information Center (NARIC)
www.naric.com
800-346-2742
8400 Corporate Drive, Suite 500
Landover, MD 20785

National Stroke Association
www.stroke.org
800-STROKES (800-787-6537)
info@stroke.org
9707 E. Easter Lane, Suite B
Centennial, CO 80112